Be Your Own Doctor

A Personal Trainer's Frustration with the
Medical Community and Her Triumphs over Adrenal
Disease and Clinical Depression

BONUS: With Fitness, Fashion and
Alternative Therapies Found Along the Way

SHIANNE LOMBARD

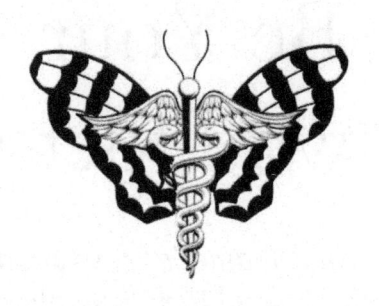

Copyright © 2017 Shianne Lombard

All rights reserved.

ISBN: 1974409708
ISBN-13: 978-1974409709

All photographs, unless otherwise stated, are strictly copyrighted to **Jessi Lynne Photography**, and it is forbidden to use the photos for any purpose without prior express written authorization from the photographer.

Cover Design:
Gina Marie Balog-Sartario, **GMB Creative LLC**

Butterfly Logo:
Designed and created by, and copyrighted to,
Eddie MacIntosh

DEDICATION

I dedicate this book to all who suffer from chronic illness, and to the families affected by the loss of a person who could once do everything and now may need you more than they ever wanted to. For me, that was my husband, Timothy Treman. He fell in love with a vivacious blonde personal trainer with six-pack abs; doing triathlons, marathons, extreme hikes were what we called FUN. As Yolanda Foster once said in a dedication to her husband, "You married me, and I fell." That episode of *Real Housewives* aired the night I lay in bed at NIH crying because I could no longer be the wife you deserved. But just like the song you dedicated to me, "Even if we can't find heaven, I'll walk through hell with you, you are not alone." You have fulfilled your promise for *in sickness and in health*. I only hope to one day find a way to show you just how much you mean to me.

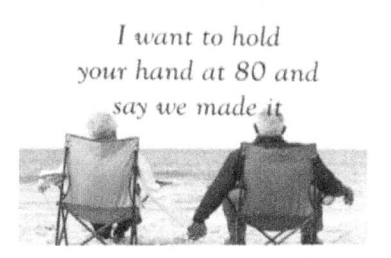

I want to hold your hand at 80 and say we made it

CONTENTS

PART ONE 8

Childhood 9

Family DJ Business 13

College Years 15

Fire 17

Accomplishments 19

Move to San Francisco 22

Tim and I Falling in Love 24

And So It Begins — Left Adrenalectomy 27

San Fran Angular Thoughts 29

Changes, Diagnoses, and Depression 31

Education about Cushing's 37

Confirmation Cushing's and NIH 40

Pre-Surgery Fun 44

Beautiful Molly 46

Surgery—Unforeseen News 49

Recovery 54

Unexplained Attacks 57

Depression and Suicidal Thoughts 62

Psychiatry and a New Road 67

Therapy 71

New Doctors and New Diagnoses 74
One-Year Celebration? 80
When Dosing Goes Wrong 80
Conversations about Cushing's 85
Finances Associated with 94
Chronic Diseases 94
Motivation 96
Food Addiction 99
Leptin, the "Satiety" Hormone 104
Ketosis 107
Reviews and Suggestions on 112
Diet and Cleanses* 112
New-Found Youth at 40! 119
Top 10 Things I Did To Succeed 121
Concluding Thoughts 124
PART TWO 125
Exercises—From Hospital to Hikes 126
Cushing's Beauty and Fashion Tips 143
Holistic and Alternative Therapy 150
Concluding Thoughts 165

ACKNOWLEDGMENTS

I would like to acknowledge every Cushie on Facebook who answered my 100s of questions when I was overwhelmed with the fear of the unknown. To Karen, the first person I ever talked to on the phone who had Cushing's (we always remember our first!). To Eugenia, a Sac and Fox Indian, the first woman I ever met in person with Cushing's (wow, they do exist!). She took me under her wing and showed me the ropes. To Caroline, my phone call the night before going into NIH that changed my entire mindset going into the four days of testing. To my editor, Maria Vano, who was with me every step of the way writing this book. She seemed to enjoy it just as much as me. I could not have done it without her. And finally to those doctors who didn't listen to me when I said something is wrong—That's right, I dedicate this book to YOU, your ignorance and laziness to do your job made me *unbreakable* for anything else that comes my way. And for that I THANK YOU. I got this.

Introduction

I want to start this book off by saying I am not an author. I am neither a writer nor reader of novels on my weekends. But I knew when everything started that it was happening for a reason. And one day when it was all said and done, it happened to *me* for a reason. I promised myself that in order for me to get through it, I had to focus outward, knowing one day I would have something to offer the world. This is my attempt at that offer and promise.

I ask you to read my story with an open mind. It's not pretty at times but it is *real*. It is not to educate you about Cushing's—you can speak to your doctor about diagnosing. This is simply what I went through and how I handled it, or failed to completely at times. I am putting it all out there for the world to see. The *good, bad and ugly*. Also, keep in mind this does not mean these things will happen to you.

Pre-diagnosis, surgery, and recovery is so very different for all of us. Resist the urge to judge or compare yourself. To question, "Why did she write that...If I wrote a book, I would have said it this way. You're not that unique." Please remember, this is my story, my therapy in a way, some of the stories may not make sense to you. It's okay—they make sense to me and I love them.

Always struggling with my health from childhood, I had to learn quickly how to feel normal, and loved teaching people what I learned along the way. I became a personal trainer, helping others to lose weight and be healthy. But somewhere along the way, I started experiencing extreme health issues of my own. My body was no longer responding to my efforts to be healthy. My appearance started to change and the things I was doing became more and more extreme as I tried to maintain a normal appearance and hide that I was sick. This book is in two parts: my life growing up, struggles, diagnoses, and frustration with lazy doctors; Part 2 is my biggest contribution. I wanted to combine my 17 years as a personal trainer with my own personal struggles to help people with Cushing's keep moving through their recovery. And be an educator to those with Cushing's, AI (adrenal insufficiency), or any chronic illness who can't just go to the local gym and ask a personal trainer—whose goal it is to make you sweat and so sore you can't move the next day. (Sorry guys, I love you but leave the tough clients to me, I kind of get it now!)

I also want to share the fashion and beauty tips I tried along the way in my desperate attempt to keep my business and livelihood going before I lost it all. In a funny way, I have no other skills, I've only been a personal trainer, and I wasn't ready to give it up. So pick a chapter you're interested in or read it straight through.

Either way, I hope you walk away with something useful, no matter your condition.

This is my journey...through Cushing's to Addison's to recovery—from triathlete to barely being able to dress myself and finally to recovering into a stronger person I never knew I was.

Join me in this walk...

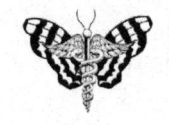

PART ONE

Childhood

For as long as I can remember, I have always loved to move. Gymnastics, working out, martial arts, and dance. Dance was my release, and I'd close my eyes and get lost in the music. For that moment, I would forget...forget about my problems, forget about my pain, and forget that I was sick.

Unfortunately, as a child I was sick a lot, seemingly forever on and off antibiotics for one thing or another, severe cystic acne, ear infections, strep throat. Acne started at age 12 and continued all the way through to college—becoming so severe it covered my face, neck, shoulders, chest, and even down my back and arms. Even with all the antibiotics, I seemed to get sick faster, easier and more often than the average person. Finally when I was 21 years old, I was given Accutane. Though it cleared up the acne for good, the damage was done to my skin, and antibiotics killing off good and bad bacteria left my digestive tract at a huge disadvantage.

Growing up in Saginaw, Michigan, my childhood was anything but peaceful. My father left when I was five years old. My two older brothers and younger sister were only 15, 10 and six-months at the time. Why did he leave? His reasoning was because his life "didn't really turn out like he wanted," having to work all the time and so on. He just wanted to live on a boat in the

Florida Keys like Jimmy Buffet. So he did. He left behind an amazing family, but one that struggled to keep their heads above water.

    My mother suffered from deep depression, and was institutionalized when I was young. My youth was spent with myself and my siblings fending for ourselves. I remember being made fun of often for not combing my hair or looking sloppy. Little did they know what was going on at home. Because of her disease, my mother looked at the world in a very skewed and negative way. Keeping her in a good mood and stable was a daily task, taken on by children and teens much too young for this—trying to cope with the stress of attempting to control our environment, while at the same time trying to grow up, was overwhelming. No child should have to deal with this, not allowed to live a carefree stable childhood. Our worries and needs took a back seat to her illness. My middle brother, Michael, attempted to hold it all together. He was forced to pay the dues of two adults incapable of following through on the life they built together. He is the reason we are all so close. He never left, never ran from the problems that were not even his, and loved us unconditionally.

    I attempted to reunite with my father when I was 21 years old. I was desperate for answers, closure, and the relationship I longed for from a father. Unfortunately, he was not capable of helping me with any of this. The conversation went pretty much like this…"Why did you leave and never look back? Why would you leave us in the care of a mentally disabled woman?" His stunning response: "Well, I figured if I left, your mother would be forced to sink or swim." When I reminded him, "But you never looked back to see if we sank or swum, because guess what? We *sank*." I asked if he ever wondered how we turned out, if we went to college, if we were happy. He concluded with, "Well, I figured one day you would find me, and see, here you are." The man had absolutely no clue, nor even remorse for leaving. Needless to say, I was devastated.

Even so, we attempted a relationship over the next year. I would call to chat, yet he seemed to always rush me off the phone. I asked several times if we could meet up again, but he always said he was working. This mediocre relationship eventually caused me nothing but more pain, so I decided to write him a letter telling him so, adding that I was hoping to be part of his life on a more regular basis. I ended with asking him to reach out if he wanted to work on our relationship. He never responded. I could not fathom a human being just walking away from his or her children, never turning back…then when given an opportunity to reunite, simply not care to make the effort. I realized then, he was more emotionally disabled than my mother ever was. But at least she sought help, while he never even recognized he had a problem. If possible, I was even more devastated than before. He passed away last year and we had never reunited. This instability and fear of abandonment would affect me for the rest of my life.

Family DJ Business

Somehow during the years, my mother was able to pull it together, and attempted to provide as normal of a childhood as she could. She tried to prepare us for the world in the best way she knew how. Fight! Yes, I mean literally fight! Martial arts. She wanted us to be able to defend ourselves in any situation. So I took up Ju-Jitsu and worked my way to earning my black belt. For some reason, I hate telling people and I don't like talking about it, but it taught us discipline, confidence, and how to take a hit and come back swinging.

My mother had always been an entertainer in a band, but didn't like to rely on other band members to put food on her table. One day she decided to go solo, combining DJing with what would eventually come to be known as this little thing called Karaoke.

She always loved to sing and wanted to incorporate that into her DJ act. She ordered cassette tapes from Nashville that had lyrics on one side and musical solos on the other. We would hand-write the words on an 8x10 laminated piece of construction paper, and people would come up to the stage to sing on a cordless microphone. This was long before a bouncing ball told you when to sing or lit up words like in today's Karaoke—we were just winging it! A female DJ back then was not a common thing, but she worked long and hard to provide for us, and I will always respect her for that. Through some of the darkest years, I watched as she lay in bed, depressed and unable to function. She would pick herself up, drive us to the show, blankly staring at the road as we drove. And for just a few hours, she became someone else. As she performed, she became an actress, pretending her life was something else. She always closed her eyes and got lost in the music—just the way I did with music and dance as my escape. I watched in admiration, not really understanding that I was more like her than I realized. She taught us an amazing work ethic, to make sure you show up when someone is depending on you, how to smile through the pain, and that no matter what you are going through, *the show must go on.* This learned skill to *fake it until you make it* became crucial in my career and illness. Given all she had been dealt, she will always be one of the strongest women I know.

College Years

I continued to struggle with my health throughout college, with odd headaches, random aches and pains, and high anxiety. Even when I was happy, I would get so excited that I would make myself nauseous. If someone called on the phone, I would talk really fast and be so nervously anxious that I would hang up the phone and have a scratchy voice and headache. If I was talking to people about fitness or something I loved, I would get so excited to teach them what I learned that I would again talk really fast, taking only shallow breaths between sentences, shrug my shoulders, and leave each encounter with severe neck pain, barely a voice left and a major headache. Another time I was so excited for my friend's bachelorette party that I stayed up all night with anxiety and excitement. When it came time for the party, I was drained, lethargic and in pain. I didn't want to be this way; it was as if I was being punished for being excited. That was so sad to me.

It was imperative for me to be diligent about what I ate and how active I was. Dance was my outlet—I was on the dance team for Spirit Soccer and Maryland's Thunder Lacrosse. I loved working out and "feeling the burn" in my muscles. Learning about the fitness industry intrigued me—I figured what better way to spend my college years than learning how to be healthy so that I could enjoy the rest of my life. After all, what's the point in making money if you don't have the health to enjoy it, right?

I graduated from Towson University with a bachelor of science in Kinesiology and a minor in Business Management. I continued on to do three internships: developing off-season workout programs in the Gilman High School athletic training department; working with Sinai Hospital's cardiac and stroke rehab center; and as a personal trainer and physical therapist aide so I could learn all aspects of the career before making my decision which direction I wanted to go. As I was working with people recovering from hip replacement or knee injuries, I felt that if I could have only gotten to them before their injury to help them gain mobility and balance, or lose a little weight before surgery, I knew their recovery would have been much easier. I decided that personal training was what I was most passionate about.

Fire

I stayed on as a personal trainer at Sinai Hospital, Lifebridge Health and Fitness, continuing to learn from some of the industry leaders until one day deciding I wanted to open my own in-home personal training business. I had it all set up: equipment, contracts, took a class on women's entrepreneurship, and had scheduled a meeting with a friend's father (an agent) to get insurance first thing on the next business day, Monday. However, that Saturday morning, just two days before I was to get insurance, I was walking away from a load of laundry I had placed in the dryer, and heard a loud boom. I turned and saw my entire hot water heater had burst into flames. The fireman's theory was that the pilot light had gone out and gas had continued the fill the cylinder. When the pilot reignited, it blew up.

You know the old warning, "Don't place items within three feet of your hot water heater"? Well trust me, they mean it! I had boxes piled up all around it, so the flames caught on very quickly. By the time the firefighters got to my home, the smoke was already rising to the ceiling. And out of an odd strike of bad luck that sometimes I think only seems to happen to me, the fire truck had done a demonstration earlier that morning at a local elementary school...and was empty of water. They ended up having to go a few streets over to hook up to a fire hydrant.

With this delay in putting out the fire, I lost everything I had worked for. I had no insurance yet and was a renter. I had run out of the house with no shoes or jacket...in January. Everything was gone. As I sat in the back of the ambulance wrapped in a blanket, a woman from the Red Cross came to bring vouchers to Walmart. I walked into the store in only my socks and picked out a pair of shoes. As I sat on the floor to put them on, I hung my head and cried, thinking "I don't even have a toothbrush, why is this happening!" Okay, time to pick up the pieces and start over...One step at a time.

Accomplishments

Eventually, I started working at Gold's Gym at the power plant as the Personal Training Director. The sales manager, Rob, was a wonderful boss and mentor in the business. He encouraged me to think outside the box and try different crazy fitness programs I had thought of. So I did! I started a new workout no one had ever seen. One day while kayaking, I realized it was an amazing workout for the core and the arms if you were paddling incorrectly. I didn't know anything about kayaking, so I just started calling local kayak companies with my pitch: "You know kayaking and I know working out, so let's get together and create a 'kayak workout'." It was a hit! People who had never even been in a kayak were signing up and spreading the word. We showed them a condensed lesson about water safety and different strokes. Sometimes we would have them switch between paddling correctly and using their core strength, then switch to arm paddling to burn out their shoulders and biceps. We ended with fun games and a great workout was had by all. It caught the eye of the local news and they had reporters out doing the workout on camera.

Then came my big break. Dr. Phil was holding a "Bridal Weight Loss Challenge." He selected six brides from all over the country. Gold's Gym is a sponsor of his show, so each location was notified and local trainers were interviewed to be the personal trainer for the Baltimore bride. Rob had me believing I could do anything, so I went for it. His confidence in me had been the stability I needed to move to new levels. I got the position! I helped "my" bride lose 80lbs before her wedding. Our story was selected to be in Oprah's magazine, "O". It was the first time I had ever been to Hollywood.

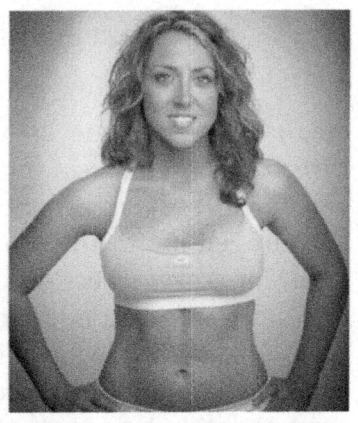

I was then selected for *The Biggest Loser*. In my season, called *State against State*, the woman selected to represent Maryland lost 107lbs! She was absolutely gorgeous. Afterwards, she met one of the other contestants on the show and wanted to stay involved in fitness. They both became personal trainers for me and together we started *Maryland's Biggest Loser*. WBAL News got involved and people from all over came to my gym in hopes of losing weight and changing their lives. We had teams and challenges just like on the show. It was a great time in my life.

I went on to accomplish four marathons, three triathlons, some extreme hikes, bouldering, skydiving, rock climbing, surfing, anything that got me moving. But still, as active as I was, I seemed to always have random aches and pains. Always seeming to take longer to recover than all the others. I kind of thought it was part of the game since I was so active, but after asking others if they were experiencing the same, I was always quite off. But I wasn't prepared for just how *off* things really were under the surface.

Move to San Francisco

Even though things were good in my life, I was having a hard time enjoying them. I still always knew something wasn't right physically. I would go to my doctor and tell him something was wrong. The downside of bouncing around from different social service programs as a child and then to different general physicians as an adult, made it hard to see patterns over the years. (Keeping your own medical records along the way is crucial.) But the response was always the same, "Of course you're tired, you're a personal trainer." So I decided to be annoying and forward and asked for a series of tests. I told him the only thing I noticed was that different doctors over the years had told me my potassium was low. Seemed like no big deal, but I did see a pattern. He ran some tests and ironically the only one that did not come back was a test for aldosterone (a steroidal hormone that regulates salt and potassium)—they had lost the test. I was so frustrated that I never followed up to get retested. Another year went by and I continued to suffer.

I needed a change and decided to move to San Francisco to be near one of my brothers. Before leaving, I visited my doctor for one last time and said, I'm moving across the country, I swear something is still wrong. I remember last year they lost a test, can we run that one again?" I had to **ask him** to run the test again!

Two days before my one-way flight to a new life, the doctor called to tell me my aldosterone was elevated by 300% and that I needed to see an endocrinologist immediately when I got to San Francisco. I was floored. Had they not lost the test a year prior, I could have started my health journey a year earlier, and it makes me wonder where I would be now.

Tim and I Falling in Love

Before I get into all the medical stuff, let me tell you about the very best part of moving to San Francisco...

On my second day there, I called my friend Ami, crying and asking why did I do this, I have no friends out here. She recommended I set up a profile on match(dot)com to meet someone to maybe just show me around. So the next day I set up a profile that simply said, "I just moved here two days ago." I explored around the site and saw a wonderfully tall 6'4" man with dark curly hair, so I 'winked' at him...and went out for the day to a double lesbian baby shower my brother had invited me to (How many of those have you been to!). When I returned home, I saw he had responded to my wink with a message, "I see you just moved here, would you like me to take you out tonight?" As a disclaimer, I would never normally have done this kind of thing! I would have spoken on the phone for several weeks and gotten more comfortable before even considering a date. But I was going out by myself that night anyway, so I thought well it'll be okay if I have him meet me at a public place and just show me around.

He was so handsome, and I got that excited, nervous feeling when we met in person, but in a city with a ratio of eight women to one man, I knew he would never settle down. So I decided to create an experiment that would end up changing everything.

At that point I had been single for several years, always letting go of a guy the minute he did something I did not like. At some point I thought to myself, I am going to be single for a long time if I always find fault in everyone around me. Looking across at him, I decided to make *him* my experiment, and learn about *me* for three months. I would simply journal every knee-jerk reaction to things he did that I did not like, focus on my anxieties created during the "is he going to call" and "is he actually going to try to get away with that" phases, and make note of all my triggers. This was all about me, so therefore I was not trying to change him into anything, least of all into my boyfriend.

Ironically, as the months passed I realized he *was* starting to change on his own! He was starting to do things that I needed, without me saying a word, and began fulfilling a much deeper need than all the superficial stuff I would have normally broken up with someone for. I always exhausted myself trying to come up with ways to manipulate and over-communicate things I wanted to change about someone. I basically did the opposite of "me." I thought I had to be tough and almost nagging to get men to change. But he was changing and it was fascinating to me. By the end of the experiment, I was hooked. This man had changed in so many ways, and at the same time I had as well. I was ALL in.

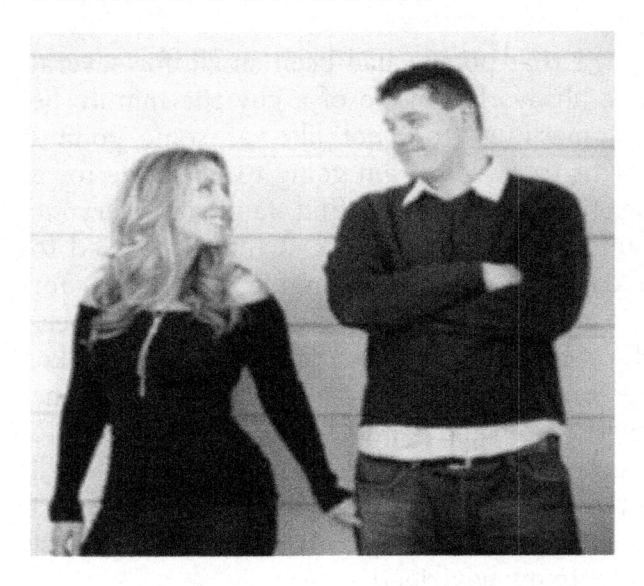

And So It Begins — Left Adrenalectomy

Back to my health stuff...I followed up with an endocrinologist in San Francisco, and he performed venous sampling* and found tumors on both adrenal glands. The results determined it was the left adrenal gland that was over-producing aldosterone (that regulates sodium and potassium). I was scheduled quickly and had a left adrenalectomy in 2009 at San Francisco General Hospital.

***Venous sampling** is a diagnostic procedure that uses imaging guidance to insert a catheter into a specific **vein** and remove blood samples for laboratory analysis.

It was a fast surgery—in the hospital overnight, rested off work for two weeks, no follow-up replacement meds, just returning to living life as normal as possible. I was really hoping to feel better afterwards, but looking back now I'm really not sure. My life was so all over the place emotionally and physically that it was very hard to tell. But deep down I knew that something was still wrong, something just wasn't right. I was continually saying to myself, "life should not have to be this hard."

Years later I would discover that several cortisol tests came back high during this time, but they did not follow up or even mention it to me, with their reasoning being: they thought they had found the problem in the left gland, and because I did not "look" *Cushingoid*. I would also later learn they may not have performed the complete surgery I was supposed to have.

San Fran Angular Thoughts

Eventually, things started getting very odd. Even though things were good, with my long family history of severe depression I knew I was predisposed. But this was something different. I could not control the negative intrusive thoughts that filled my world.

For example, I drove a scooter in San Francisco. As I would drive down the road, my mind would almost play a screenshot of a high-speed chase, like a car coming out of nowhere and hitting me. I would then picture how my body would hit the ground, what bones would break, and the angles at which things would fall. It would happen so fast, I never saw it coming. I'd try to continue through my drive, then another flash of an accident. My shoulder would twitch as I pictured it hitting the ground. Then my knee would jerk as I pictured my legs being trapped under the bike.

Another time, I was sitting at a café with a friend having a regular conversation, my eyes were looking forward, smiling and laughing at her story, but my mind was elsewhere. Suddenly I pictured the thick wood beams of the ceiling falling in on us, what angle they would fall, what bones or muscles would be injured. Again, it was always angular or geometrical and very gruesome.

Sometimes I would experience what felt like a "brain skip" or "pause." It's hard to describe, but it would seem as if my brain stepped away for a second or two, as if I was looking at my life and talking but someone else took over. I called my brother Michael in Maryland and said, "I truly think I'm going crazy, something is wrong."

I always considered myself a happy-go-lucky person, but these thoughts would come into my head, almost as if I got slapped in the face. I would continue on with my day and try to shake them off. But some days they fired relentlessly and I was not able to fight them. I wanted to just give up and go to sleep.

I allowed myself to cry. And cry hard. A release of sorts. I was no longer in control, nor did I know how to fix it. I remember thinking, wow, my mother always talked to us about depression and how your thoughts can take over, but that does not mean they are real. I could see how if someone who was going through this wasn't familiar with depression, they would think they really are going crazy and do something rash. But I knew better, and tried to seek help immediately. I explored different medications, some making me feel strange, others making me feel no emotion at all. Finally, one that targeted those types of rash thoughts for me was *Prestique*. How could this be? How could a drug change the way you think? I didn't care; I just knew I felt a little more back to myself.

Changes, Diagnoses, and Depression

One year, while visiting home during the holiday season, Tim asked to see some Baltimore real estate. I was hoping for a fixer-upper as we looked around seeing what Baltimore had to offer. But the minute he walked into the model homes of a brand new community being built by Ryan Homes, he was sold. Had it not been near my friends Rachel and Brian, I probably wouldn't have considered it. We spent that New Year's Eve signing papers and picking out what color hardwood floors and granite countertops we wanted! It hit me...wow, okay, I guess I'm moving back to Baltimore. So in 2013, after four years in San Francisco, we decided to move to Maryland to build a home and start a new life. Of course this would entail selling my old business, all of our belongings, moving across the country with just a few boxes of clothes, starting a new personal trainer business in Baltimore—not to mention planning a long distance wedding from San Francisco to be held on the east coast. Crazily enough, we landed in Baltimore on May 1, 2013, with our wedding and house completion scheduled for May 31! The wedding took place in an amazing beach house on Bethany Beach, and of course our home was not ready exactly the day it was supposed to be—so we spent the first three weeks of our blissful marriage living at the Best Western truck stop. But Tim always has a way of making the best of things!

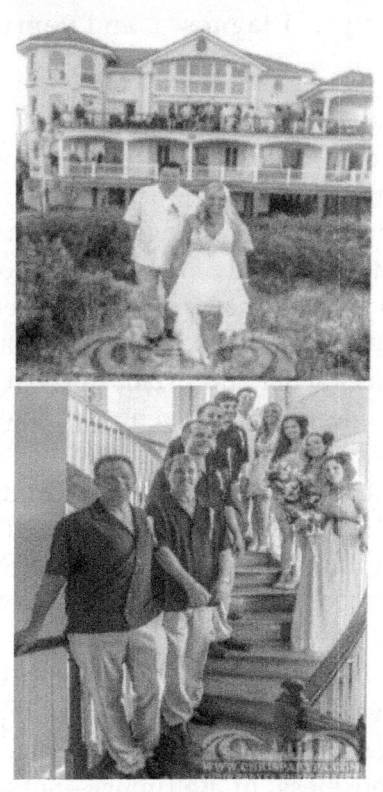

We did it, though! After getting married, we decided to try to start a family, so I started paying more attention to my cycle. I noticed my periods were very irregular, stopping completely in 2014. The post-wedding and moving back home highs slowly went away, and reality set in. Things seem to deteriorate very quickly that particular year as I slid into a very deep depression.

I had been chasing individual symptoms, but it didn't really occur to me that they were related back to adrenal. As I said, I didn't feel better either way after surgery. But they had told me there was a tumor on the other gland, so I thought I should look into it. I was determined to make it my New Year's resolution to make an appointment with an endocrinologist. It really is an exhausting task to tackle your health—doctor appointments, testing, blood work. You need to be in a good mental state to follow through and keep pushing. However, I was chasing each individual symptom, never knowing they were all connected. I found an endocrinologist in Baltimore, who immediately started the basic blood work, which included an initial cortisol blood test at 8am and a dexamethasone suppression* test. Both came back extremely elevated, with no suppression.

*An overnight dexamethasone suppression test checks to see whether dexamethasone suppresses (changes) the level of cortisol in the blood. Normally, when the pituitary gland makes less adrenocorticotropic hormone (ACTH), the adrenals make less cortisol. Dexamethasone will suppress levels, helping to diagnose Cushing's in determining the over-production of a tumor.

He sent me to Johns Hopkins, where they ordered a plethora of tests, several 24-hour urine collections, blood tests, and dexamethasone suppression. I couldn't believe it—all the Johns Hopkins tests confirmed something I had never heard of before: Cushing's Syndrome. Being told I had a rare disease threw me into an emotional state that overwhelmed me, and I just kept asking "How can this be? I'm a personal trainer who focuses on her body!" I left the doctor's appointment in disbelief. I truly thought they had no idea what they were talking about, so I pretended it didn't happen and went straight to the gym for a client. I tried focusing on my client, but couldn't. I went in the back of the gym and started crying. It was scary to me that I didn't understand what they had even told me. The words they told me were brief, quick...flying around my head trying to make sense of this—I had already had an adrenal gland removed! Then something about having the only remaining adrenal gland removed. Being on steroids the rest of my life. Carrying around an emergency injection, and something about a Medical ID bracelet. It was so confusing; I was losing control of my body and mind.

Things progressed again very quickly. The depression worsened, and I would spend hours in my bed, sometimes not getting up until 4pm. If you're familiar, depression is debilitating. You cannot describe it to someone who does not suffer from it. Depression hurts and it is *real*. Ironically, my years of watching my mother fight to get through days, never giving up and always "putting on a good show" became my reality. I didn't have a choice. My career—and livelihood—was on the line. I would rest in my car between clients, set my phone alarm and pray that when I woke up, I would feel just an ounce better. But there were days I remember barely being able to stand long enough to shower—with my eyes closed as the water rushed over my face, I would talk to myself, "just lift your arms to wash your hair, come on, you can do it, just lift your arms to wash your hair." It was all I could do to stay standing. How could I go from marathons and triathlons to barely being able to wash my hair?

Each small task became a chore. I was annoyed and edgy often. Every hour, I waited to see what ache or pain my body was going to throw at me, and what pill or breathing technique I would use to get through...or would I just cancel my day and retreat back to bed in the way I watched my mother do for years? Every hour was spent weighing and measuring my energy and pain. If there was an event, I had to plan ahead. Ibuprofen or Excedrin? If I use too much Excedrin before the event, then it won't work when I really need it to. I have a bit of energy now but if I go too hard, I will pay later and get sick. Day in and day out I watched as my body fell apart: muscle started deteriorating, hair was coming out in chunks, period stopped completely, always pain in my digestive tract, my midsection was growing and I was gaining fat in odd ways. I was embarrassed. I stopped telling people I was a personal trainer and hung my head if I saw someone from my past. This loss of control of one's body and mind is the worst hell one can ever go through.

One day while at the gym I had my hair in a ponytail and I looked at my side view in a mirror. There I saw a huge hump on the back of my neck. Oh my God, was this the "buffalo hump" they were referring to? For anyone unfamiliar with

Cushing's, a *buffalo hump* is a pad of fat that forms between your shoulders at the base of your neck (or sometimes in front). They say this accumulation of fat at the base of the neck and midsection is the body's way of protecting the vital organs and brain stem since the body is in crisis mode from over-production of Cortisol—the stress hormone, better known as *fight or flight*.

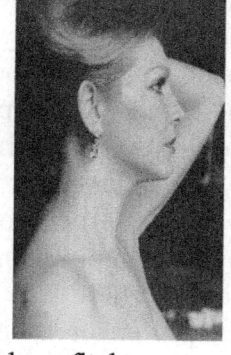

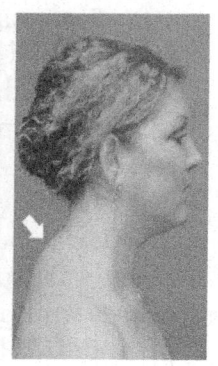

    I again ran to the back of the gym and broke down in tears. It was devastating for my ego. For me, I had always used my body as the way to judge my success as a personal trainer. It was my livelihood. I had to hold it together because I wanted to lead by example. But now I was embarrassed by my body and it was something I could not control...and that was the hardest part of it all. I spiralled downward into drugs, alcohol and food addiction, anything that would get me through, if only for that moment.

Education about Cushing's

This is general information found on the web about Cushing's. I don't want to go into too much detail because the disease affects everyone differently. Plus there is Cushing's Syndrome (adrenal) and Cushing's Disease (pituitary).

Cushing's disease is caused by a pituitary gland tumor (usually benign) that over-secretes the hormone ACTH, thus overstimulating the adrenal glands' cortisol production. *Cushing's syndrome* refers to the signs and symptoms associated with excess cortisol, usually due to tumors (usually benign) on the adrenal glands causing over-production of cortisol. Cushing's syndrome can also be caused by a producing tumor located ectopically, most times found in a lung (if not found on an adrenal).

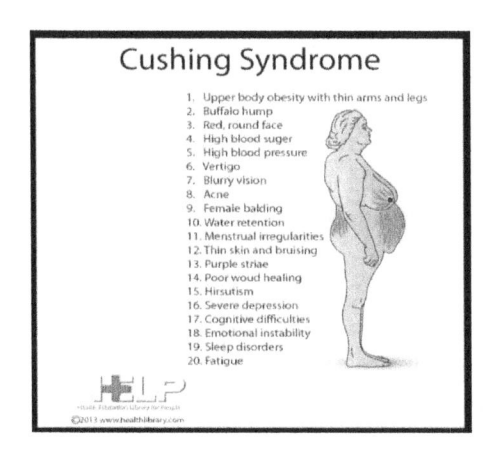

Cushing Syndrome
1. Upper body obesity with thin arms and legs
2. Buffalo hump
3. Red, round face
4. High blood suger
5. High blood pressure
6. Vertigo
7. Blurry vision
8. Acne
9. Female balding
10. Water retention
11. Menstrual irregularities
12. Thin skin and bruising
13. Purple striae
14. Poor woud healing
15. Hirsutism
16. Severe depression
17. Cognitive difficulties
18. Emotional instability
19. Sleep disorders
20. Fatigue

The ***adrenal glands*** (also known as *suprarenal glands*) are small endocrine **glands** located on top of each kidney. They produce a variety of hormones including adrenaline and the steroids aldosterone (to regulate your sodium and potassium) and cortisol (your stress hormone, also known as "fight or flight"). Each **gland** has an outer **cortex** which produces steroid hormones and an inner medulla.

An ***adrenalectomy*** is an organ-removal surgery that removes one or both of your adrenal glands, along with the producing (or non-producing) tumor. The adrenal glands are two small organs, one located above each kidney. They secrete hormones that help regulate many bodily functions, including your immune system, metabolism, blood sugar levels, and blood pressure control.

Laparoscopic surgery, also called *minimally invasive surgery, band-aid surgery,* or *keyhole surgery*, is a modern surgical technique in which operations are performed far from their location through small incisions (usually 0.5–1.5 cm) elsewhere in the body.

Post-Surgery Sick Day Rules. According to NIH, sick day rules for patients on steroid replacement (hydrocortisone, dexamethasone, or prednisone/glucocorticoid), present dosages should be increased as follows:

- ✓ If your fever is 100.4°F or higher, double your dose;
- ✓ If your fever is 102°F or higher, triple your dose;
- ✓ If you experience vomiting and/or diarrhea, then double or triple your dose depending on severity. Take a double dose for mild to moderate symptoms and a triple dose for severe symptoms.

There are standard tests normally used for diagnosing Cushing's (I had them all):

> 8am blood test
> 24-hour urine collection
> CT Scan (for adrenal)
> MRI (for pituitary)
> Dexamethasone suppression test
> ACTH test
> Midnight cortisol blood test
> Saliva Cortisol test

Confirmation Cushing's and NIH

I always jokingly say that Facebook saved my life. It's all about who you know, and you never know who will change your life forever. That time came when my friend Chuck brought me to an annual boat party. I reunited with Diane, an old friend. Ironically, after celebrating her bachelorette party, several of us became friends on Facebook. Now, again I will preface this story to say I don't usually friend someone right away after meeting them. But Karla, one of Diane's friends, was so nice and we all wanted to exchange the pictures we had taken, so of course we became friends on Facebook.

Well, that's when it happened. A few weeks later, I put out a post asking if anyone out there had ever heard of Cushing's. Karla, whom I had only met at Diane's bachelorette party, responded and said her sister works at NIH with children with Cushing's. She immediately put me in contact with the right people...ahhh, the power of the Internet! Like I said, it's about who you know. You never know when someone can come into your life and change it forever. See, I don't think I would have ever been convinced I had Cushing's after a couple random blood tests—I needed something more extreme to convince me.

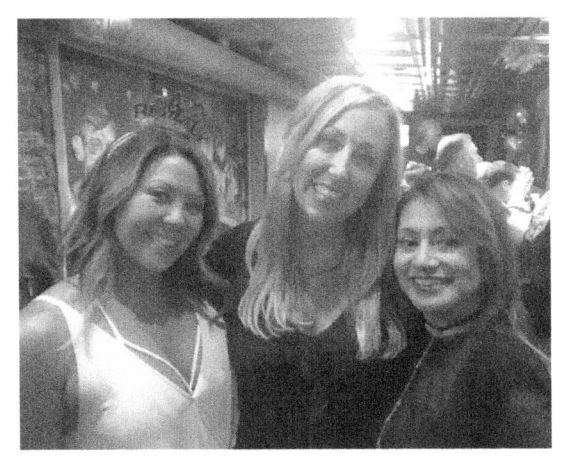

Before going for a scheduled four days of testing at NIH, I made a special trip to Los Angeles to meet with Dr. Friedman. He is a Cushing's specialist who allows Skype, phone or email appointments after an initial in-person consultation. He confirmed the Cushing's elevated cortisol numbers.

I then went to NIH for the four days of testing, meeting first with Dr. Stratakis, who was confused by my numbers. He said, "We will have to see for ourselves. You don't look like you have Cushing's, but your numbers are extremely high" (my 24-hour urine Cortisol was 425, on a normal range-scale of 5-50). They said they wanted to run their own numbers for verification.

A few days before I went in for testing, I spoke with a woman online who had been to NIH for Cushing's testing. Her tests came out inconclusive because she was what they call

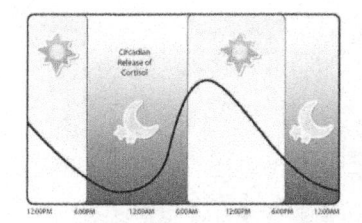

Cyclical Cushing's. She went another two years before she was actually diagnosed and had tumor-removal surgery. That one phone call with her changed everything—suddenly, I wanted to have Cushing's. Strange, right? But if I did, then that would mean it wasn't all in my head.

NIH uses several blood, urine, and hair sampling tests. The nurse said she was only going to take a small section of hair the size of a pencil tip. I figured, okay, she would yank a couple pieces out, no big deal. She went to the crown of my head and began twisting my hair tightly. As she showed me the clump of hair, I screamed; it was thick as a pencil, not pencil tip! Come on, I had already lost so much hair, now you're taking more! (Later, when it grew back straight up like alfalfa, I could only just laugh.)

NIH also uses a *midnight Cortisol blood test* to confirm diagnosis. You must "fail" the midnight cortisol test as well as at least four of the 12 tests to be considered Cushing's. I failed all 12 tests and my midnight cortisol was 17 (normal range 0-3). What this means is that even at midnight, when your natural circadian rhythm should be at its lowest in order for your body to rest and repair, a person with Cushing's overproduces cortisol at all times; thus never allowing the body that absolutely necessary rest and repair time. This is why we have all of the random complications and side effects for nearly all aspects of our body. *(Image ©t-nation.com)*

The doctor and nurse came in at the end of the four days of testing with the pronouncement, "It's confirmed you have Cushing's." I fell over onto my pillow from where I was sitting on the edge of the bed, as the nurse bowed her head and softly said "I'm so sorry." I sprung back up laughing and said "NO! I'm happy! It wasn't all in my head!" The doctor said, "Well then congratulations young lady, you have full-blown Cushing's (*AN: there are other types, pseudo, cyclical, florid*). You've managed your symptoms well. You're the healthiest sick person we've seen." I danced around in a circle and said "Thank you! That is the best compliment anyone has given me as a personal trainer!"

I then asked what I thought was an innocent question: "I don't know if I want the surgery, it sounds so scary. Can I just continue to live with the tumors and attempt to manage all the horrific symptoms?" He said, "No my dear, your levels are extraordinarily high." When I asked bluntly how long I would have, he responded, "About five years." I stared blankly at him, like my mom used to stare at the road while driving. After a few moments, he said, "I know this is hard, but you have your answer, stop searching. Haven't you suffered enough?"

Pre-Surgery Fun

My surgery was scheduled for two months later. With all of the fears that come from receiving information-overload, I decided to just LIVE for those two months. I didn't know how my life was going to change after surgery. I didn't really understand how someone could function without a vital organ we are all born with.

So I decided to go all out...I planned a trip to Mexico with my husband and friends Costi, Diane (who got me into NIH) and her husband Donnie, along with crazy nights out with girlfriends (you know who you are), and special time spent with my family.

For New Year's Eve we had some friends over. Standing at the high bar in our kitchen, I had a grand idea to have everyone lean in at the bar for a selfie. As we all positioned around to fit, my neighbour Matt yells, "Shianne, you're on fire!" My hair had caught fire from a candle I had on the bar. Boy it went up fast with the gallons of hairspray I had used! Come on, I had already lost so much hair being sick, NIH took a huge clump and now it catches on fire! Boy, this was a rough start to 2016.

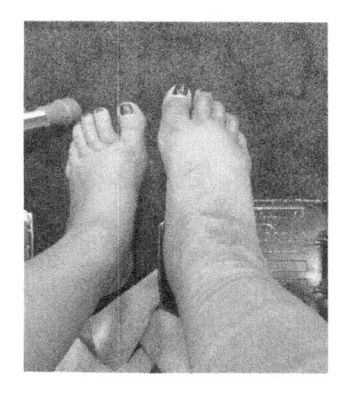

I definitely went a little crazy. During a bachelorette party for my friend Marissa, 17 of us celebrated in Vegas. I ended up breaking my ankle the very first night I was there and had to use a knee scooter for the rest of the trip. But it wasn't going to slow me down, no way—I just scooted around to the pool parties and out to dinner at night! The girls were so supportive and made it fun. When I got home, I was placed in a large black boot. It was challenging to personal-train and move around like I was used to, but I had to just accept it.

All of this taught me a lot—that I am a bit of a spaz. I rush everywhere I go. If I have a thought, I rush up the stairs before I forget it. As soon as I think of something, I spin around, knocking things over to get to whatever was so important at the time. This all changed with that boot. I had to learn to do things SLOW. I never realized how hyper I was until I was forced to slow down. Ahh but it was all part of the plan, helping mold me to adapt to my new norm.

Beautiful Molly

The weekend of my husband's birthday, we had decided to celebrate it in Ocean City with our friends Laura and Rich. We had left our two adorable Maltipoo dogs (siblings) with a dog sitter whom we had used several times before. Unbeknownst to us, though, the dog sitter's pitbull had just given birth to puppies. As a protective mother, their pitbull attacked our 8lb female Maltipoo. She bit down hard, fracturing Molly's skull and snapping her brain stem from being shaken back and forth. However, in order to protect their dog, they lied to us, saying Molly had had a seizure and hit her head on the dog bowl tray.

It was one of the worst times of my life. Molly couldn't walk or move, and wasn't even able to stand to relieve herself. She just lay there, limp, unable to wag her tail or lift her head. So my husband and I would lay a trash bag on the bed between us—if it happened in the middle of the night, we would both jump out of bed, he would wash her in the shower and I would reset the bed. We were a good team like that.

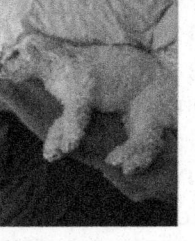

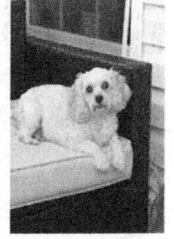

We paid for her to get an MRI...$2000! Ironically, it was the same day my insurance denied me an MRI on my broken ankle from Vegas. I actually took her to the same place I would have gotten mine...I jokingly thought, since I'm paying $2k, can't I just stick my ankle into the MRI machine with her, or maybe climb in there with her, holding her and oh look is that my ankle?! Sorry, just had to laugh in the middle of the chaos.

Lying between us in bed one night, she wiggled over to me as I was sleeping. I awoke to be nose to nose with her as she licked my face and her tail began to sway. With tears in my eyes, I knew just how much of a fighter she was, and that things were going to be okay.

So here we both were, not in control of our bodies and not quite sure what our future health would look like. Slowly she started lifting her head. The neurologist said as long as she did something new every day, she was on the road to recovery. I would time how long she would hold her head up, at first 10 seconds, then 20...eventually she was able to stand. Baby steps! Little did I know how often I would use those words.

Well I'm happy to report that Molly is 98% recovered! She still loses her balance often but runs and plays with her brother, Charlie, like nothing ever happened. I guess we all have a little fight in us—even with things that originally seem insurmountable.

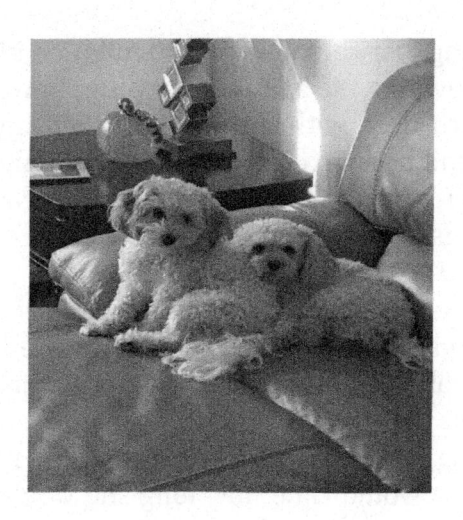

Surgery—Unforeseen News

A short time before surgery, I received a call from NIH. They said the scans showed that I did not receive a full left adrenalectomy in San Francisco back in 2009. He said the surgeon had left a part of the gland behind. WHAT? I was in shock. How could this be? When you go to a hospital, you expect to have what they told you was going to happen, a full left adrenalectomy. I called my endocrinologist in San Francisco. He, too, was confused. He said the surgeon didn't make any notes stating he left some behind. I called my mother and sister and before I could even get the information out, I went into a full panic attack, hysterically crying and hyperventilating, screaming at them, "I can't do this anymore, I don't know who I can trust!" My sister softly said, "Shianne, I don't think it's healthy to be in this state of anxiety going into your surgery. You really need to be of sound mind to be able to handle what's to come." I went back to the doctor's office to do what I needed to make my current situation bearable.

On February 1, 2016, I had my right and only remaining adrenal gland removed at NIH.

I got up the morning of hospital admittance, did some last-minute laundry and housecleaning so the house would be clean when I returned. At one point I do remember feeling a little lightheaded and dizzy. Other than that, I was laughing and joking with my husband and nurses as I got settled into my room. I made fun videos for my friends and just for my journal the night before my surgery. Sometimes I would just talk...talk to my phone camera about whatever I was feeling at the time. Just before going into surgery, I made one more funny video. I had changed into my gown, showed my viewers the great room I was in, and apologized for any videos that followed under the influence of the awesome pain meds I was about to experience. I don't know if it is my coping mechanism or just the way I am, but I always need to find the humor in every situation. Laughter is therapy!

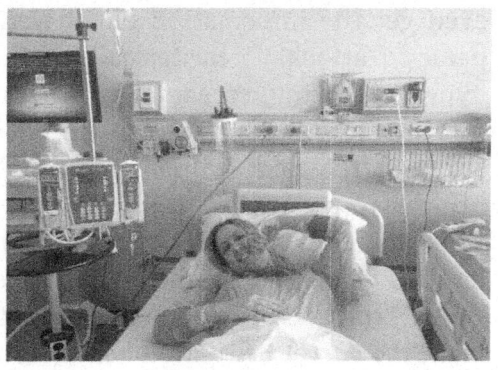

The surgery was robotically performed and went well, however somehow my liver was accidentally clipped, causing a little added pain and bleeding. It was cauterized, but necessitated being in ICU for the first three days. My mother, sister, and husband were there when I awoke from surgery. "I made it," I said with a groggy voice and blurry eyes. My husband kept asking the nurses, "Is she in pain, please make her comfortable, I can't stand to see her in pain." Below are the tumors and removed gland.

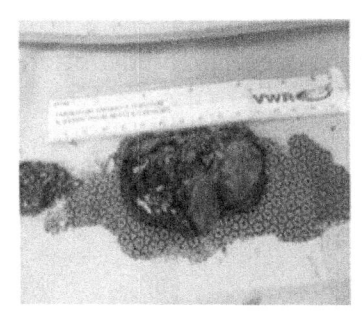

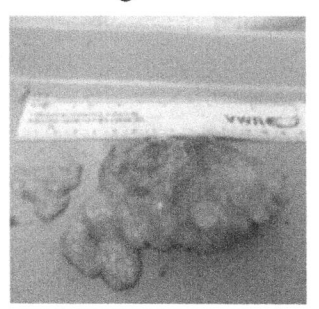

As long as I stayed ahead of the pain and took my meds on time, I was okay. One time I fell asleep and missed a dose, waking up in horrible pain. I found setting a timer to be an excellent solution, and suggest it highly to stay on track.

On the second day, I remember the nurse coming into my room in the ICU saying, "Okay, you have to walk down the hall just a few feet and back to your bed." I looked at her like she was crazy—I couldn't move, didn't she know that? My husband was there, so with him holding my hand and me leaning on my IV pole, I shuffled along like an elderly woman. A few nurses were passing by and cheered me on as I slowly passed by. They knew it was my first walk after surgery and how challenging it was. It actually felt great to move, but someone had to push me to do it (hey, kind of like a personal trainer!). Moving your body is the best thing you can do after surgery.

NIH nurses taught my family and me how to administer an emergency injection of *Solu-Cortef*. I failed a few times, but my husband was a pro. Thank goodness! Never did we realize how often he would have to put those skills to use.

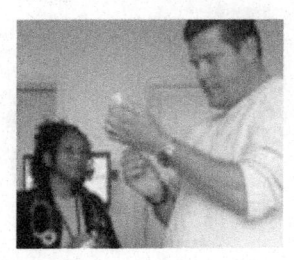

I spent a total of eight days at NIH adjusting the pain medications up and down. More fun videos were made under the influence, with me singing to the camera and making funny faces. Sometimes it wasn't so fun, as the pain meds would just knock me out, and I would feel heavy in the bed, but others allowed my pain to be tolerable, and I was able to walk around. They encouraged me to walk around as often as I could. It is the last thing you feel like doing, but is very helpful to recovery. With the right medication, they urged me to walk slow laps around the floor as often as I could. Once I did five laps! I was so proud of myself...who knew a triathlete would one day be proud of a few laps. And not because I was recovering from some cool athletic injury I did while attempting some new extreme sport, but because my body no longer could. This would be my new norm.

A couple suggestions for hospital time:

The nurses have so much to do, but you must stay on top of them. Also, bring your own bendy straws for the hospital and later for home use. That way when you take your meds you don't have to sit all the way up to sip your water since you will have four or five abdominal scars from surgery.

It's nice if you have a family member there to help understand when doctors come in to explain your progress and keep your meds on track. You are on heavy pain meds, so you may not remember all the details and questions to ask.

As I mentioned, you won't want to move, but push yourself to do it. Moving your body is the best thing you can do after surgery, and you will feel much better.

Also, your digestive tract is very sluggish after surgery, and pain medication often causes constipation. Plan some light soups to eat the first few days. Do not splurge on pudding and sugar given to you by the hospital (a personal pet peeve of mine). This is the time your body needs all it can to heal.

Recovery

Anyone will tell you everyone's recovery is different. I was told the body takes the first year to adjust to its new normal, and things tend to get worse before they get better. But they *will* adjust and you *will* get better.

I took about one month off of work after I got home. People think that personal trainers work out with every client, but this is not the case. We can choose the level of activeness for each client that we are able to do at the time. My clients were wonderful, they were glad to have me back, and very supportive of my recovery. Ironically, it ended up motivating each of them. They knew things were an extra challenge for me but I showed up. They started coming more regularly and not cancelling because they were not in the mood or had a headache. They were more motivated and consistent than ever.

The first two weeks I just rested, getting up to walk as often as I felt up to it. Around week four, I attempted some light yoga-type movements at home. Anyone watching would have thought I had never worked out a day in my life. I couldn't hold a pose to save my life! I was a bit discouraged but decided to find and grab the positive out of it. I thought, wow, now I know what my clients go through who've never done yoga. It gave me a whole new experience and perspective that would help me empathize with my clients.

Since everyone's experience and recovery is so different, I would read other people's stories and wonder why my body wasn't doing what I needed it to. It made me angry at times. I lived a healthy life, and didn't even drink alcohol until I was 28 years old. I worked out regularly—I was supposed to benefit from all those good deeds. I was a personal trainer!

Although I can honestly say that even though my recovery was horrific to me, there are so very many people who suffer way more than I did. But you know what? I do believe my health put me in a better spot than if I had never worked out before. I urge everyone to get as healthy as you can <u>before</u> surgery! Your recovery will be much smoother.

As I mentioned earlier, soup is a wonderful way to get the nutrients you need to recover, and is easy on the digestive system. In addition to my recovery, for some unknown reason the muscles in my jaw locked shut. I could only open about an inch. Thankfully, my friend Desiree had organized our group of friends to bring me soup on different days. Des has always been so thoughtful through the years, kind of the mama bear of the group, but little did she know just how crucial those soups would be to my recovery. My friends also created a group text message that we used to communicate. If I needed something, I could text the group and whoever was available would respond. This was a comforting option that I ended up having to use more than I could have imagined.

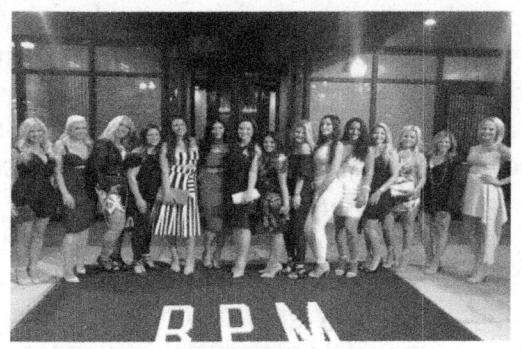

My girls!

One day I was resting on the couch and all of a sudden it seemed as if I had been jolted by a lightning bolt. I jumped off of the couch, going into a panic attack. All of the chemicals in my body were changing and adjusting to no longer having this high level of cortisol in the system. I had been told I would experience "Cortisol withdrawal." NIH tapered me quickly over the eight days in hospital, and I was discharged on 25mg of Solu-Cortef (hydrocortisone). The withdrawal was no joke. I had bouts of crying, random muscle and joint pain and emotional breakdowns. I became a pro at doctor appointments and blood draws. I wondered if my body would ever recover.

Unexplained Attacks

About two months after my surgery, it started. The one thing I feared the most...the unknown, the one random side effect that they had never seen before. I started experiencing very odd attacks. My day would simply start out normal, then I would start feeling tired, my arms would get very heavy, my eyes would lower, glaze over and become glassy. Eventually the muscles in my face would droop and my voice would change to a low pitch. My breathing would slow. Each word was an effort to speak. Soon I would not be able to hold up my head or open my eyes—though I could hear everything around me, I couldn't respond.

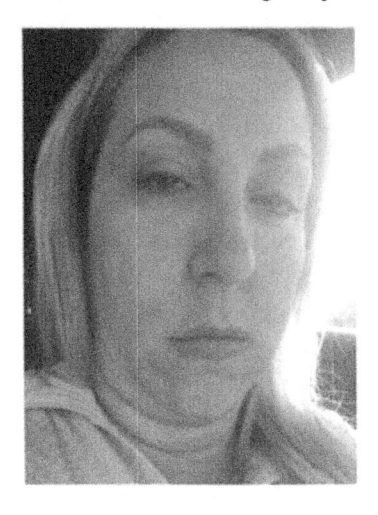

I thought it was an adrenal crisis. They educate us about **adrenal crisis** before we leave the hospital, so I just assumed that's what this was. I would *up-dose* (meaning to take an extra dose) my steroid or use my emergency Solu-Cortef 100mg steroid injection. In less than an hour, I would feel better. However, when I would go to the emergency room after each injection, the doctors would say, "this doesn't quite fit the explanation of an adrenal crisis." I didn't know what to say; all I knew is that I had never experienced this type of attack before my adrenal glands were removed, and that when I up-dosed my amount of steroid I felt better. I didn't know the worst was yet to come.

Over the next year I suffered over 100 attacks, up-dosing and adjusting my steroid accordingly. I would go to each doctor, show a video of my attack (that I had had the foresight one time to hit the video record button on my phone as it began) and ask what was going on. This actual video footage was crucial. What is this attack? How is it that everyone is saying it is not an adrenal crisis, yet it never happened before I had my adrenals removed, and when I take a higher amount of steroid it seems to pull me out. I was told the steroid is often a band-aid. It can mask and mimic several other underlying conditions.

One day I had an attack while training a client. My husband could not get across town to me fast enough to administer my injection, so the paramedics were called. On the stretcher in the back of the ambulance I could hear the medics confused on what to do with the Solu-Cortef. Remember, I cannot respond or move during the attacks but I can hear everything. The medic had to make three different phone calls for permission and a walk-through on how to administer my shot. The intramuscular injection works fast to bring me out of the attack. I later asked the paramedic why it took so long to administer it. He said "Well, you're considered an ICD-10" (I'm pretty sure that's the term he used). I asked what that meant. "Well, they taught us this stuff in school but said you were too rare and that we probably would never see this out in the field," he laughed. "Now I can tell my class I actually saw an ICD-10!" Really? Well I'm glad you didn't take too long to make those three calls, as it could mean someone's life. Officials are trying to get laws and protocol in place with regards to EMTs, paramedics and the administration of emergency injections. Please check with your local office to learn your state's rules. You may be surprised.

Moving on, my energy between attacks was lacking, if non-existent. I felt like I had taken an Ambien sleeping pill and had to go about my day in this daze and brain fog. I would find my eyes closing when I would drive, and would slap myself in the face and reposition to try to stay alert. It felt like what I've read narcolepsy is like, of a sort. But no amount of sleep would help me feel alert.

I don't drink coffee, so I have no tolerance to caffeine. But someone told me about a five-hour energy shot which would really change things for me. I didn't like drinking them (and don't think everyone should drink them), but just two or three sips would change my mood and my brain function. There was something in the ingredients I responded to very well. However, everyone is different.

Almost every day I would need to take 800-2400 of ibuprofen or Excedrin migraine due to some pain or headache (it worked well because of the combination of aspirin, which thins your blood, and caffeine which makes it more potent).

I also tried Adderall. Of course, all of these gave me energy, but I knew they were just stimulants. For a person who would not take an aspirin for a headache her whole life, I was now reliant on pills to get through my day, sometimes taking over 30 pills just to get through. I didn't think I was asking for much—I just wanted to be able to get through my day, enjoy my clients, make a little dinner and not want to feel like I was on a tranquilizer all day. I would cry to my mother, "Why is my life so hard, why can some people get away with not being healthy and never have a single headache or random ache or pain?" Yet all my efforts seemed to just frustrate me more that my body would not cooperate. I had never worked harder at anything with little-to-no results. I wanted to just feel good naturally, without a stimulant and pain medication.

But sometimes that wasn't an option. One night, those 30-plus pills taught me a lesson. As I sat in a restaurant with Lindsey, I suddenly got nauseous. As she was driving me home, all the pain killers, steroids, Florinef, aspirin, caffeine, and anything else I needed to just get through my day, all met and went to war in my stomach...then all over the side of Lindsey's car and down O'Donnell Street. She just calmly drove me home, and helped me into my house as the attack was coming on. I flopped on the couch as she picked up my legs and positioned my head to make me comfortable. She got my steroid to up-dose and we waited. Lindsey never wavered once, staying totally calm (well, except for fumbling to get the pill bottle open and a hundred steroid pills flying into the air like confetti), but even that did not phase her. She just made a joke and continued to patiently care for me. It is always a challenge for friends to watch you be less than you once were. Challenge for them, and you.

Depression and Suicidal Thoughts

You would think that the **attacks** would be the most challenging part of recovery, right? But it was getting through that and making it to the other side with my mind and emotions intact that proved the most challenging. Part of cortisol overload is the messing with emotions and the inability to control them—they don't just disappear with tumor removal. The after-effects of this nightmare disease/syndrome are massive and long-lasting, creating a whole new part of recovery. Unfortunately, I was now dealing with extremely negative intrusive suicidal thoughts. No actions or tendencies, but the thoughts were very real to me at the time. My negative intrusive thoughts were not like the odd angled thoughts I spoke of earlier while in San Francisco. This was more along the lines of...I would see a large house, and while the average person would think, "Oh I wish I had a large house like that," and maybe self-reflect with "I don't work hard enough to have a big house" and move on to the next thought. But not me, no...mine would continue with thoughts of "You're worth nothing, you've done nothing with your life, you're worthless, life is not worth living, you should just kill yourself!" The thoughts would just pop into my mind, come so quickly that I couldn't prepare myself for such negativity. I would stop and shake my head as if to shake the thought away, continuing down my path or whatever I was doing that day. Just as I calmed, with no warning another negative intrusive thought would come, then another. It was exhausting.

One time I was walking through a store with Tim. There was this nice fuzzy blanket that was similar to one his mom had. I said to him, "Oh look, a fuzzy blanket like your mother's," to which he innocently commented, "Yeah, that's really nice but I'd want a different color." We continued walking down the aisle and my mind would start. "That was a stupid comment to say the blanket was fuzzy, your husband thinks you're an idiot. Know what? You ARE an idiot, you've done nothing with your life, he wants a divorce, you should just kill yourself." Are you kidding me? All that from just saying that a blanket was fuzzy.

One weekend we were in Rochester, New York (where Tim is from) for the Easter holiday. He always called it "the center of the universe." I loved going there. The six-hour drive in the car was wonderful, talking about absolutely nothing with my husband and having our two dogs with us, music blaring and the convertible top down. Life doesn't get much better than that. But this day was particularly hard; I kept thinking negative intrusive thoughts as we drove, picturing trucks crashing into cars. Trying to have a playful conversation with my husband became a little more challenging. That night I was lying in bed thinking of how hard life had become and thoughts intruded of ending it. My husband joyfully walked into the room holding our beautiful Molly puppy that was the joy of our life. "She wants to kiss you good night," he playfully said. As he pretended to dance with her across the floor, I immediately put on a smile, pretending like I was okay for that minute, and kissed on her for a moment. As he walked out of the room, I collapsed back down onto the bed and continued my negative thoughts of ending my life. It was sad because I wanted to be so much more for him. He's never known what happened that night...until now.

But here's the thing—you can have everything going for yourself and still suffer depression. I don't think I totally understood that until now, and it's very interesting to me as you always hear of Hollywood stars dealing with depression or even suicide, and you wonder why. I never fully understood the depths of how a chemical imbalance could literally take your life, and no one or nothing can pull you out.

At the same time, I knew that, yes, we all get down or depressed during certain circumstances or stressors in our lives. But strangely, it was at this point that I considered my life the least stressful it had been in a while. I mean, really—I had a wonderful husband, was getting along with my family, my career was going well (even though I was unable to make as much money as I wanted), we had a beautiful home, two amazing pups…and yet I struggled with depression and negative intrusive thoughts. So all of these factors can affect anyone, no matter the situation. But even so, I kept thinking I was going crazy, saying to myself, "It hurts too much to live, I want to be strong, but honestly if this is life then I just don't want to play anymore. It's just not worth it to me."

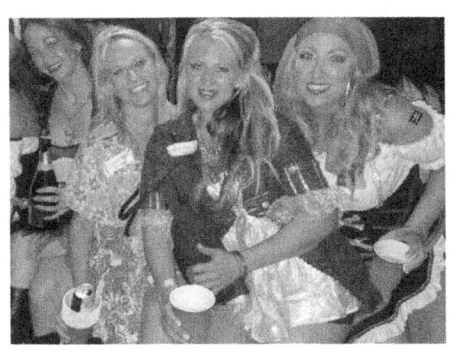

I would call my friends to cry (you all know who you are). Sometimes I wouldn't even know it was coming. I was making a healthy dinner one night, talking to my friend Lindsay on the phone. She asked simply "What are you up to tonight?" I said, "Oh, just trying some new healthy recipe because I have to be good, you know." As I pushed the vegetables around in the pan suddenly with a little harder push, I said again, "I've got to be healthy," with added irritation in my voice as I gradually got louder until I screamed out, "Because, you know, if I don't THEN MY WHOLE F*CKING WORLD TURNS UPSIDE DOWN!" I threw the spatula across the room and grabbed the pan, slamming it to the floor. I continued yelling, "*I*

can't do this anymore, Lindsay, do you hear me?! I just don't have any fight left in me!" I sobbed uncontrollably, I couldn't breathe, and all I could do was hold myself in a ball, rocking back and forth on my kitchen floor surrounded by my food. Neither of us saw it coming. Lindsay let me cry, waiting until I caught my breath, not trying to come up with something clever or helpful. She just listened. Eventually she lightened the mood and we began to laugh. That's the thing—sometimes all we need is to vent. Scream. Cry. Tell your family members or friends what you need from them in these moments. Most people just want to fix you. This will simply frustrate you since they can never fully understand. They will tell you, "Just be happy you're still alive." Please don't waste your energy trying to make them understand. They *are trying*, and sometimes people say inadequate things.

I give these examples, again, not to say they will happen to you, but only to say you are not alone. You are not crazy. But it's better to know you may experience things like this so it's not so scary if you do. You will fall, but you WILL get back up—each time with a scar that will toughen you for things that 90% of people couldn't think to handle. Your only choice is to fight through it. Recognize when you need help, recognize when you need a break, and recognize when you just need to feel sorry for yourself and cry.

Psychiatry and a New Road

It was time to do something, this couldn't continue, it was too strong. During one of my emergency room visits, I was lying in my hospital gown talking to my friend Ami. I needed help and knew it was time to ask for it. She told me to reach out to her friend Arman, a psychiatrist. I knew him from the gym back in my six-pack ab days, but I was too embarrassed to let him know I was sick. My hands were shaking when I dialed his number. I tried to play it off like it was no big deal, but then realized people can only help you if you let them. I told him my doctor recommended I find a neuropsychiatrist, and he said he had just the person in mind. He made a personal phone call to Dr. Crystal Watkins at Sheppard Pratt. She was not currently taking new clients but he asked if she would do him a personal favor. I am to this day so happy that she agreed, because I knew in our first session she would be the therapist to walk through this with me. We went through the long list of previous medications I had tried: Prozac, Wellbutrin, Zoloft, Trazodone, Xanax, Clonazepam, Effexor, BuSpar. All with some pros and cons, but nothing that stands out. Paxil made me unable to cry, literally unable to feel. Prozac made me numb to life and not care about anything. Prestique, as mentioned earlier, definitely helped with the weird angular geometrical thoughts I had in San Francisco, but that was not my issue anymore. She listened about my attacks and Cushing's. It wasn't that she was an expert on Cushing's, but she was willing and excited to help me piece it all together. And that was all I needed.

I told her my symptoms and how much I was struggling with negative intrusive suicidal thoughts. She explained that lithium was the best treatment option for suicidal thoughts. I had always had a stigma against lithium for some reason; to me, that's what they gave people who were manic and going crazy. Funny how I didn't put myself in that category no matter how bad things got, so I declined and continued on with other options.

Then came the night I was with a client and the thought came into my head for the first time, "Tonight might be the night I end it, I can't do this anymore." There was nothing going on that night or that day that had upset me, so this was a random, matter-of-fact decision my head seemed to have made. This scared me tremendously. Realizing that those thoughts are only momentary thoughts that change rapidly and frequently, I held on to this and refused to get caught up in it. The next morning I was at the doctor asking to be placed on lithium.

Within two weeks my life changed. No more negative suicidal thoughts! I couldn't believe how much it helped. How could a pill change the way you think? It didn't matter, though; I felt better and wondered why I had waited so long to get help.

A few suggestions that helped me: I was always very sensitive to medication (one Benadryl and I was knocked out for days) and realized then that I had a low tolerance. When I would start an anti-depressant or new medication, it would make me feel weird and "out of it," so I would stop. My mom taught me to ask for a *pediatric* dose of any new medication. I would start slow; though it might take a week longer to feel the effects, it was well worth it.

I also learned to give each medication time to do its job. Some work within weeks and some can take months. Give each medication three months before you decide if it is working. Track how you feel each day so you can give feedback to your doctor.

If you do choose to come off a medication, **never** stop all at once. This is your brain chemistry we are talking about. Even knowing this detail, I have still weaned too quickly and paid dearly with odd withdrawal symptoms. One time, I thought I was weaning off Latuda correctly; oddly enough, my lower jaw started involuntarily jerking painfully from side to side. I didn't even think about the Latuda, though. I went to my trusty Cushing's Facebook group and asked for opinions. Someone responded with an article about withdrawal symptoms from Latuda.

I was shocked—I blamed it on my Cushing's withdrawal, when it wasn't. Never underestimate the power of the Internet and Facebook!

I encourage anyone who deals with emotional instability to please get help. Do not hesitate. Cushing's messes with the mind and emotional state, and whether you're pre- or post-operative or even just starting the journey, what it does and has done to the emotions is sometimes very hard to deal with. Sometimes you will start to feel better and think you can come off replacement or other meds. You may still be very fragile. It's kind of like when you break your arm and start to feel better. You think you can take on the world. But have someone barely bump or bang that arm and all your old feelings of pain may return. Your determination to "not go back there" must persist. Discuss everything with your doctor and loved ones. Your emotional state and wellbeing is crucial to your ability to handle all the ups and downs of surgery and recovery. You must be clear-headed to make good decisions about your future. The stigma surrounding psychiatry and therapy aside—this journey is hard enough to deal with on one's own—your mental health is the most important.

Therapy

It's important, though, to find a therapist with whom you connect. Try different ones until you find a good fit. It is crucial to talk through all of the emotions before, during and after with someone who is objective. Through my friends Marybeth and Becky, I was lucky to have found my therapist, Dr. Long. I always go on referrals from friends; online reviews are good, too, but nothing compares to a friend's recommendation. Remember: it's great if you find someone who understands your condition, but don't waste tons of time looking for only that. Try a few and see if you connect. Most importantly, ones with whom you connect and who are willing and excited to work with you.

Dr. Long made me look at things in a whole new way, correcting me if I subconsciously said something that was all or nothing. Phrases like, "I will never recover" become replaced with "I haven't recovered yet." We used CBT (Cognitive Behavioral Therapy), which is a short-term, goal-oriented psychotherapy treatment that takes a hands-on, practical approach to problem-solving. Its goal is to change patterns of thinking or *behavior* that are behind people's difficulties, and so change the way they feel. He also explained to me that I was basically suffering from a form of PTSD (Post-Traumatic Stress Disorder), because the cortisol level in my body was raging non-stop for years, naturally becoming so high that my body, muscles, organs and brain thought I was always in crisis; therefore, deep neuro-pathways were formed that had to be broken for the cycle to subside.

Looking back, I was always very outspoken, saying exactly what was on my mind with no real filter. But as my life and the disease progressed with bizarre thoughts being some new norm, all of a sudden I had a sense of a filter. I'd pause before speaking, wondering if each thought was real or due to a particular state of mind. Let's face it, no one needs to know each and every odd thought running through our head at all times! I realized that my emotions and mood were only determined by the chemical balance or imbalance in that moment, and not based on the situation but how I felt right then and there.

For instance, if I'm singing to the radio thinking fun thoughts such as my book release party and suddenly someone cuts me off in traffic, I might shake my head and think, "Well I guess you're in much more of a rush than me." But if I was imbalanced that day, feeling extra stressed and with lack of sleep, I would scream obscenities to the driver, getting myself more worked up. Nothing changed in the situation, each driver cut you off, but your reaction was only based on your chemical mood at the moment.

We've all heard how soldiers home from war react at each loud bang, the body reacting with increased blood pressure and heart rate, muscles tense, chemicals start pumping to get ready for what's to come. Though he or she might be able to see it was a car or a balloon and there is no danger, the body is still reacting. Eventually after enough time goes by and work is made to control those automatic noise reactions, different neuro-pathways will be created, and cortisol returns to the natural momentary fight or flight response (***momentary*** being the keyword). But it takes time and work. This is crucial to recovery.

New Doctors and New Diagnoses

With all of the various issues and "undecided" opinions about what was going on, I made a decision to switch endocrinologists, and reached back out to Karla, whose sister worked at NIH, and asked for a referral. She recommended a new one in Washington, DC, Dr. Susmetta Sharma, who specializes in Cushing's and its after-effects. After just a couple minutes of listening to her, I knew she was the doctor for me. She explained to me that oftentimes after treating Cushing's (the producing tumor), other ailments can surface. That many times, the high level of cortisol suppresses conditions; once the cortisol returns to normal, it no longer suppresses and they resurface. She said the attacks could be presenting as a neuromuscular disease or even Multiple Sclerosis. I was floored. I couldn't believe that throughout that entire last year, over 100 attacks, increases of my steroid...and it was not an adrenal crisis as I thought! It was all wrong. How could my previous endocrinologist let me go a year without helping me figure these attacks out? Guess it was time to <u>be my own doctor</u>, piecing together each detail from each specialist. I knew then that no one was going to care as much about my health as me.

I came home and took a long walk around the neighborhood, going over everything in my head. I didn't know much about MS, just that it was a debilitating disease that often ends in a wheelchair. The thoughts again of how could this be happening to me, how did no doctor pick up on it, whom can I trust, this is my life we are talking about, how does no one know what's going on…all spun around in my head.

As I wandered, I saw my friend Zam was home. I frantically called him and said, "I'm coming over, have a vodka shot ready." He stood stunned as I paced in his kitchen, screaming at him, "How could they be wrong? Why is this happening to me?" We took another shot, and he desperately tried to find the words to console me, but what does anyone say in a moment like this? I recognized his heartfelt effort and knew there was nothing I could do at that moment but to breathe.

It was St. Patrick's Day, and I was meeting Lindsey and Bella to celebrate. As I got to the crowded Canton Square, it was not the time or place to share the news with my friends. So I pretended it wasn't happening, trying to forget all the doctor had said. I was doing pretty well until I ran into two of my neighbors, Hillary and Courtney. Joyfully we celebrated together with another shot. Hilary innocently asked, "How are you feeling?" Within seconds my emotions ran wild, and I broke down in tears, hysterically crying on Courtney's shoulder in the middle of El Buffalo. They both tried their best to summon the right words. I pulled it together, realizing there was nothing I could do at that given moment, so I turned to my friends and said, "Tonight, we forget."

I was alone the weekend I found all this out because Tim was away. The next night, I broke the news to Bella, who, not wanting me to be alone, did some research online and immediately came over with burritos! This may seem like a little thing, but it was so special to me—someone other than my family cared enough to research my condition and help me put the pieces together. I will be eternally grateful to her for that night. She had even found a video on YouTube showing various MS attacks on her phone, and as we watched them and others, all I could do was think, "I'm not alone." I'd never seen anyone going through a similar attack. But...as we slowly opened other videos, we came across one very disturbing attack. As the seconds passed, anger grew in me until it became rage, screaming "NO!" as I realized that might one day be me. I threw my burrito at her phone, rice flying everywhere and collapsed over on the table's bench, bursting into tears. It was a long night for Bella.

This was the lowest time for me pre- and post-surgery. I can honestly say that I gave up, going into what I call my survival mode. I allowed myself to do whatever I needed to get through the day. If I was in pain, I took ibuprofen (thank goodness I never got into the harder pain killers), if I was nauseous I took Ondansetron, if I had a headache I took Excedrin. I hit a downward spiral into drinking and drugs, partying to numb the pain. I needed to step away and reboot. This was my darkest time.

My endo scheduled me for a follow-up MRI that revealed white matter lesions which can represent MS—but one of the reasons why Cushing's is so hard to diagnose is that it can mimic several diseases. Unfortunately, at this point the damage was done. Because I had up-dosed so many times to either treat or prevent a "crash" (that's what I called the attack because I looked like my body just gave up and crashed out), I had now given myself what's called *steroid-induced Cushing's*! I still had other Cushing's issues, the buffalo hump, a "moonface," random aches and pains that had gotten worse, gained 40 pounds, and wasted a year putting my body at risk with high steroids. Doctors have a tendency to blame it all on stress, or say it is psychological. Do not allow them this easy out. Granted, stress is "a silent killer," but you know your body better than anyone. No one ever quite determined exactly what those attacks were, but after seeing seven neurologists and five endocrinologists, along with seven days of overnight seizure monitoring, they have classified it as "non-epileptic seizures." The search continues.

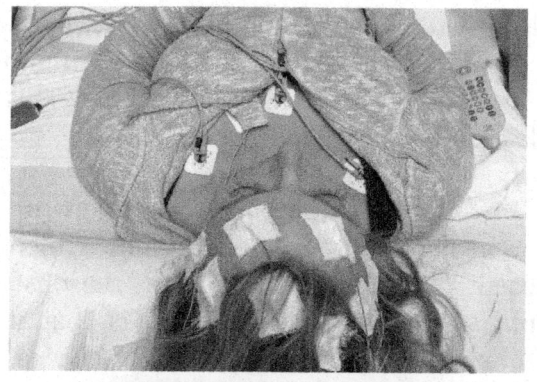

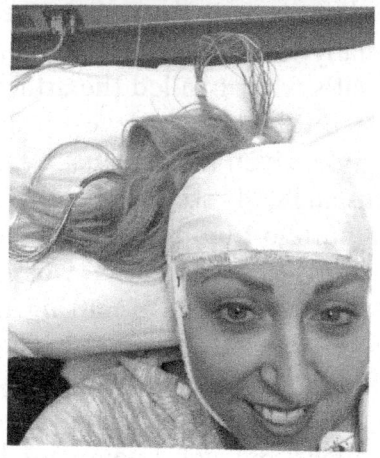

So once I was told the attacks were definitely not adrenal crisis, I was advised to not take an extra dose of steroid the next time one occurred. This was very scary to me because they still did not have a true definition of what the attacks were. All I knew was that the steroid would pull me out of that state, and without the up-dose, didn't know what would happen. All I could do was try to live my life and continue to see clients...Waiting for the next attack. Talk about anxiety-production!

Inevitably, as I knew it would, one day it happened. Grabbing my phone as quickly as possible, I called my husband, who could always tell by the tone of my voice that I was having an attack. He came immediately and rushed me to Johns Hopkins emergency room, where they monitored me throughout the crash, for the first time without an increase in steroid. This was terrifying to me. Even though they told me it was not adrenal crisis and not to take the steroid, they really didn't know what it was. So what if I go into this comatose state where I am unable to move, speak or lift my head and I don't come out? Is it okay for my body to be in this state for hours where I can't breathe normally and my central nervous system just shuts down? All we could do was wait it out and pray for the best.

It lasted eight long hours. At about six hours in, I was able to open my eyes and look around and lift my head; by the eighth, I was able to sit up and shuffle around. Blood test, blood pressure, EKG, all were normal. I had made it through my first attack without additional steroids.

One-Year Celebration?
When Dosing Goes Wrong

In the circle of "Cushies," we call these "brainaversary" (pituitary brain surgery) or "andrenaversary" (adrenalectomy). When my one year celebration came, I wanted to have a party to thank all my clients, family and friends for standing by me. I had it all planned out in my head before, because I just knew that by the time a year had gone by, I'd have blown through recovery, lost all the weight and would feel amazing. Wrong! It couldn't have been further from the truth. I was still dealing with the unknown attacks, was sick the entire week before with the flu, and had gained 40lbs!

I was trying to do things that would make me feel good, so one day while shopping with Lauren, as we stood in line at the Towson Mall, I glanced across the shoe store at my reflection in the mirror. I gasped and stormed out of the store. Was that *me*? I didn't even recognize myself! Lauren was confused—everyone told me they didn't see the moonface and puffiness. Like others, she tried so hard to say the right thing. And she truly meant it. But I was in a head space that could not see what others saw. She knew my plan was to feel amazing by my one-year anniversary. But like they say, "God laughs when you say you had a plan."

Once I'd gotten my emotional state stable, I was no longer doing any up-dosing for any reason, getting to (what we call "weaning down") 15mg. My range had been 15-20mg. However, over time I learned that 15mg was too low for a bilateral adrenalectomy. With no adrenal glands, the body is no longer producing, and being on replacement steroids is a lifelong necessity. The correct dosage is crucial and is worked on with a knowledgeable endocrinologist (who is hopefully Cushing's-specialized), who orders tests every six or so months.

One day I had woken up with a strange feeling, not really able to pinpoint anything but knowing something just didn't feel right. Being stubborn, I continued getting ready to meet Rachel and Michelle for a spin class at Merritt Athletic Club, where I had been the Personal Training Director before I moved to San Francisco. I was wearing a heart rate monitor...that showed a rate of 172bpm before I even began spinning! I sat on the bike with no tension, barely pedaling. After a few minutes my left leg started to tremor. I told my friends I was going to leave the class early and would meet them outside. As I stood up, both of my legs started to shake. I tried to rush to the door to get out of the classroom, when all of a sudden my long keychain rope got caught on someone's bike. It yanked me back, and, because my legs were shaking, I fell to the floor, face first, legs and body tremoring similar to a seizure. I could hear everything going on around me, people yelling, "She's having a seizure, move the bikes!" I heard Michelle and Rachel desperately trying to remember every random thing I ever told them about Cushing's, but I was unable to respond. Someone called the paramedics. Rachel and Michelle attempted to gather the class away from the paramedics to give me privacy. I asked Rachel to cover my face with a towel so no one could see my expression. I was embarrassed and ashamed. Here I am in the gym where I had once been the Personal Training Director, lying on the floor incapacitated. I was placed on the stretcher with my legs strapped down, and suddenly went into another seizure-like state. The paramedics stood with their bodies lying over my legs and body, fearing my vigorous shaking would tip the stretcher over. This was particularly scary because the tremors were new, instead of the normal lethargy and inability to move. I frantically yelled "RACHEL" and she rushed over to hold my hand. "I'm here babe" was all I needed at that moment. She handled it like a champ! It is hard for any friend to watch someone go through this, but they never made me feel ashamed or embarrassed. The next day I jokingly texted them, "Wanna go to spin with me tomorrow?" I figured I probably wouldn't be invited to another spin class anytime soon.

Another time, as I was training a client, we had been sitting on the floor for a bit and were getting up to move to some machines across the gym. As I stood up, it felt like every bone in my body needed oil, as if I were compressed and couldn't stand upright. As my client continued to walk, I was near frozen, unable to move properly. I pretended to play with my watch as I shuffled toward her, bent slightly forward. I was so embarrassed and wondered how much longer I could hold down this career. It was my passion! I had so much knowledge and desire to keep helping people, but how could I if I couldn't get my own body to cooperate? It was sad in a way...the ultimate irony.

All of these things were signs that my dosing was now too low. I had gotten it wrong again. I ended up being taken to Johns Hopkins and had a plethora of tests and blood tests. The results were astonishing—potassium was dangerously elevated (6.6, with a range norm of 3.5-5.0), sodium was extremely low and out of bottom range, magnesium was very high, I was dehydrated and my kidneys were barely producing. The consensus was clear—taking the steroid down to 15mg was too low, and my body needed the minimum of 20mg. This was along with Florneff, which I'd previously been at 0.5 and was increased to 1.0mg. So many things had been happening due to not enough steroids, and now throughout recovery and for the rest of my life (or anyone having no adrenals) it would be a constant maintenance of the correct level. Cortisol is essential for our bodies, hence the fight or flight, and the regulation of other functions (blood pressure, heart, kidneys, etc.), but too much or too little, and trouble reigns! And now, I've experienced both.

Conversations about Cushing's

With all the ups and downs I experienced, I realized no normal person would understand what I was going through. I had to adjust my expectations for every person in my life. Not to say they didn't love me, but just because it was all I could think and talk about didn't mean they had to. I learned that I couldn't rely on just one person—it would be too exhausting emotionally for them. That's when I realized I needed several different support systems and people in my life I can call, and not just placing the entire burden on my husband or family members. They love you, but are often not equipped to always say or do the right thing. They desperately want to make you feel better, but they may not have the tools to fully understand what you need in the moment. Just be patient and know they love you more than you will ever realize.

Attempt to educate them. If you find an interesting article, copy and paste just the area you want them to understand the most. They may not take the time to read the entire article, but if you keep it short they might absorb it. Lead them to reputable websites such as CSRF (Cushing's Support and Research Foundation); because if they start searching "Cushing's" on the internet...well, you know how crazy that gets. My mother tried searching about surgery for Cushing's and bombarded me with fear that they were going to "cut me wide open" instead of laparoscopically. She worried herself, calling me at all hours about this random fact she read on some obviously outdated website and could not focus on anything else I was trying to tell her.

Ask what your loved ones need from you. Both pre- and post-Cushing's you'll have limited energy, and many times you must choose where to put it that day. For instance, I asked my husband, what do you need from me as your wife when it comes to the house? I was nearly floored when I listened as he told me that to him, a clean kitchen meant there were no dishes in the sink. Why was this so surprising? Because for eight-plus years, as I wiped the counters down, cleaned the appliances, and scrubbed the stove and floors, he never seemed to notice. One thing I did all the time, routinely, was place all the dishes in the sink as I was cleaning the counters. It was always the last thing I focused on (I grew up with dishes in the sink all the time). So here I am thinking I'm doing a good job cleaning the kitchen every day and wondering why he doesn't notice, when all along he is irritated by the dishes in the sink. So there I had it, I could put the small energy I had into doing the dishes first, instead of everything else first—he is happier, and I don't feel a constant guilt that I'm not doing enough.

In the same way, tell your loved ones what you need from them. If you just need to vent, say it—but before you start so they are not consumed while you are talking with thinking of all the suggestions they are going to give you to *fix* you. They will be more than happy to just listen with no pressure.

Repeat yourself. As I said earlier, people will ask questions that you have answered 100 times before, even to that same person. Resist the urge to feel they are not listening or that they don't care. This is *your* obsession. Hours spent online trying to understand it all has left you edgy and tired. It's okay, they don't have to understand everything. They just have to love you, and so far they have been pretty good at that. Give them a break.

Most people don't understand Cushing's because of its symptoms. They don't understand what you are going through. They want to help you, but have no idea how; wanting to say the right things without having the tools. It's like trying to describe childbirth to someone...unless you go through it there are few words to describe the impact it has on your life. Be patient, though, and concentrate on the effort they are trying to make even if the words do not come out correctly.

Speaking of words...remember, women use far more words than men ever will. Women are wonderfully emotional and detail-oriented. We often over-talk things and men (or anyone, for that matter) may only absorb a portion of what we are trying to say. Please allow them to do it wrong a few times, wait and reflect on it. Then, at a totally separate, non-emotional time make positive suggestions for the future.

If you're lucky, you will have that special someone who may not be in your life as much as you want, but when they speak, *watch out!* For me, that was Lena—friends for over 10 years, she always had insight about life and a way of explaining the dynamics between the brain and the body. Her wisdom amazed me. Even though she didn't suffer from Cushing's or anything close to it, she got it...she understood. She had been through her own struggles and empathized. She was able to put thoughts and feeling into words and make sense of how I could handle any situation. She challenged me to look at things in a totally different light, talked me down off the ledge a few times, and possibly saved my marriage a few nights (I'm kidding about that one, of course!). I can say most people are not like Lena. They are not deep and introspective. They may ask odd questions, maybe the same questions you've answered a hundred times. It's okay—be patient, explain it again. "Yes, the adrenal glands are located on the kidneys. No, not the thyroid, that's in your neck, your *kidneys*."

Then you have those people who just want to help. Surround yourself with these people, ones who push you and influence you in a positive way. My friend Dani followed my journey closely. She always called to check in and wanted me to talk to her friend Lydia to get on vitamin supplements and hormone replacement. I was wary at first, but she kept after me, gently mentioning it each time we hung out. Lydia was indeed a wealth of knowledge. They both took a personal interest in *my* wellbeing, and truly just wanted to see me happy.

The core of my support system:

My husband: Coming from the dysfunctional upbringing or lack of a father figure, one of my proudest accomplishments is that I have found and maintained a healthy, loving, and trusting relationship with my husband for almost 10 years. After all I have been through, I can say I was set up for disaster, raised to hate men, yet somehow found the most caring, loving, amazing man I will ever know. He is all I will ever need from a partner, and I am honored that he chose me to walk through this life with. My friend Lena always says, "If you meet Tim and you don't like him, it's *you*."

My elder brother, Michael: Now this is the most ironic person to have the biggest influence on my health. Long brown curly hair past his shoulders, usually an unkempt beard, and dirty torn clothes from the car he has just worked on or house he just fixed. Probably the most unlikely source of better living through nutrition. He and his wife, Sue, listen to health podcasts all day and are really into food and natural medicine. With the stress of our family, he wasn't the warmest brother growing up, but more along the lines of: "Call me if your car breaks down, but otherwise I will talk to you at Christmas." Recently I haven't been able to get this man to stop calling me...several times a day he checks in on me or tells me about something he and Sue learned online. He hounded me to get healthy and try the Colorado Cleanse (I talk about this later). Initially I didn't want to do it, but one day he asked me to take a ride with him, just the two of us. He said we were going to do this together, changing the way he himself ate so he could understand more about what I was going through. I was so touched. He DID love me, in his own way, and I had misjudged him for years. He had also urged me to schedule a phone call to a doctor in California he followed, to get his take on the attacks when I was at my wits' end and had given up—yet again Michael came to my rescue with his persistence to get healthy.

My younger sister, Dani: Second to my mother, one of the strongest, most resilient and amazing women, mother to six (yes, six, including twins—Caleb, Alaina, Juliana, Jeremy, Aaron, Ashlyn) whom I have ever met and I'm so very blessed to call her my sister. Danielle's belly laugh is contagious. She truly lives in the moment and takes on the world as if nothing can stop her. She stood by me every step of the way, taking notes, spending hours researching my disease online and asking doctors lists and lists of questions to make sure she didn't miss a thing. I am in awe of her every day.

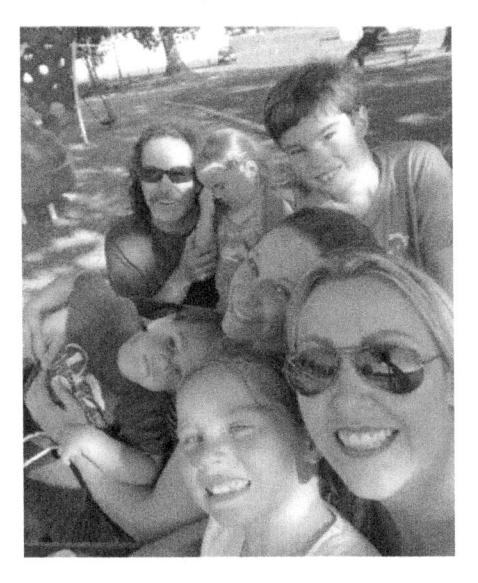

My mother: Although she struggled with her own demons, I wouldn't be who I am today without her. She would always say, "If you don't ask, the answer will always be no." I rolled my eyes as a teen but have now come to realize I have to ask questions, I have to be persistent—if not, my life is on the line. It's a shame wise words of parents are thrown to the wayside until they one day define you.

My best friend forever, Nina: I always say Nina is who I want to be when I grow up! Her grace, undeniable friendship, caring personality, and beauty inside and out. This is the type of friend you know you can always rely on and who will go out of her way to make you feel special. She was the first woman I met in San Francisco, and we've stayed friends and will remain friends until we are sitting in a rocking chair one day reminiscing and making jokes. So I basically got a husband and a best friend out of San Francisco. Wow, thanks San Fran!

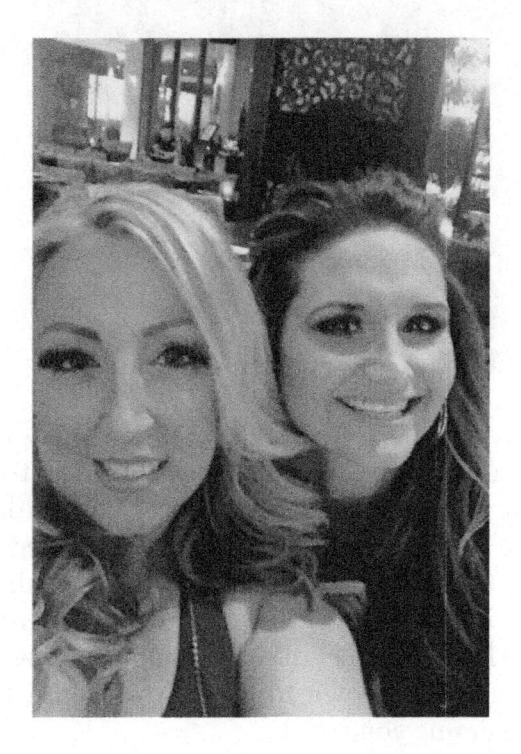

At the end of the day, support system or not, always have a goal or something to strive for! Create an interesting life you're excited to talk about when you see friends and family. Your support system doesn't have to be a group of people. It can be a pet, a particular park or location where you feel safe or that brings back good memories. A warm blanket or comfy pyjamas that just feels good against your skin. This is your support system.

However, on the flip side, remember that when people start getting healthy, family and friends are not always supportive and this can be extremely hard to deal with as you're trying to make it through this thing called recovery. This surprised me, but I truly think it's because people simply do not like change. Suddenly your family and friends feel resentful that you are able to make changes in a healthy way, but it affects their time spent with you. Now going out for dinner is not as sinful as it once was when you commiserated together. It's hard to believe, but sometimes they try to sabotage your progress. Be aware of this and choose wisely with whom you surround yourself during this fragile time. If this kind of thing is happening, remember that therapy can also help you as you make this transition.

Finances Associated with Chronic Diseases

Financial stress places stress on any healthy person, marriage or family. Plan ahead for your medical bills; learn about your insurance plans and how much deductibles will be. The first year of all the health issues, we were bombarded with bills, and even with great coverage a trip to the ER was about $300. This year we chose a plan with a high deductible and 100% coverage after it's met. I recommend choosing the high deductible if you can for the first year while you may be figuring odd things out. For me, I'm now at a point where I'm stable in recovery, everything is set and so we will go back to regular 80/20 coverage next year.

To gain some insight into financial issues and insurance, we took Dave Ramsey's *Financial Peace University* and is usually offered through many or most churches. They have all dates and locations on their website. He says you must attack your goals with "gazelle-like intensity" because though a cheetah is faster than a gazelle, it will many times get away in a chase. Why? Because its life depends on it! You must be like a gazelle and attack each of these issues as if your life depends on it—because it does!

BE YOUR OWN DOCTOR

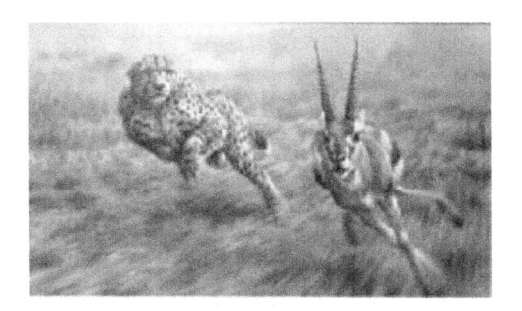

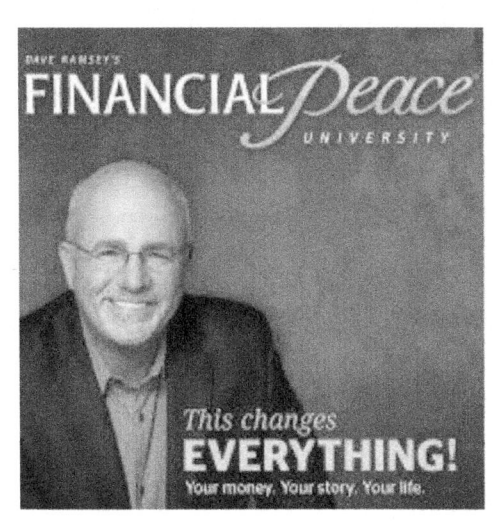

Motivation

Along the way I was asked to write an article describing my struggles for the Cushing's Support & Research Foundation (*www.csrf.net*), established by a community of researchers, physicians and laypersons. While this is still considered a rare disease/syndrome, there is much research being done to spread the word and increase both medical and layperson knowledge. We can beat this fatal disease! One night I received an email from someone who had read my article. I was astounded by what I was about to read:

> Hello Shianne, I just finished your article...I think it might have saved my life. Last night, I just couldn't ask God for any help anymore, because I felt like everything in my body was rapidly deteriorating. I was getting up from furniture like a 90 yr old grandma. I am 56 & I had my left adrenal gland removed. No physician informed me at all about the recovery. As of 2 days ago, the depression became paralyzing & the "negative intrusive thoughts" became relentless & unbearable. I was convinced that other things were going on, & that any hope for a quality life was over. I felt like I had a nervous breakdown, & it was my end. I suppose that is the level

that people reach when they take their own lives. Any sense of reality is completely shut out. How could Dr.'s leave all of this info out? It's outrageous that this procedure is treated w/such ignorance.

Anyway, God bless you w/all of my heart, because before I read your article, I was convinced my life was over. My deepest apologies for laying all this on you from a complete stranger. I realized there is something very effective in reducing the deep level of recurrent depression episodes in order to regain a proper prospective & realize that there is a wonderful world out there for me, but at the time, my mind cannot see it for anything.

This email motivated me to write this book. I knew I had to give back. Not only suffering through the physical side but also the mental. As I said earlier, I was taught about depression and still thought I was going crazy. It makes me cry to think of all who suffered who were not familiar with what depression felt like, and especially if their doctor did not inform them of the chemical changes Cushing's brings. I want to fight to bring awareness to an unknown and often misdiagnosed disease, to reduce the years sufferers go through shuffling from one doctor to the next, from the GP to the endocrinologist to the neurologist and back again. To have pill after pill be given to them in an effort to control all these symptoms. And finally to help people, family, friends, doctors, nurses, personal trainers or any health care professional identify the signs and symptoms, and stop the eternal chase after each individual symptom, never knowing they were all related. From Cushing's to Addison's Disease to the average person dealing with adrenal fatigue, we must all educate ourselves and others on this crucial organ sometimes considered our "second brain," due to all that it regulates. Arm yourself with knowledge.

CUSHING'S DISEASE
http://cushingsmoxie.blogspot.com

IT'S TOO RARE.	MAYBE EAT LESS.	SURE. UH HUH.
What DOCTORS say	What FRIENDS say	What FAMILY says
IT'S YOUR FAULT.	IT'S THE TUMORS.	CUSHING'S KILLS. GET HELP.
What SOCIETY says	What PATIENTS say	What YOU should know

Food Addiction

Hunger is a temporary form of insanity

I want to preface these sections of food addiction to say Cushing's does **not** cause these things, although the Cushing's impact on the imbalance of chemicals and hormones may exacerbate any condition that existed before. Because I was in the body/food-focused fitness industry, I was predisposed to having challenges in these areas more than the average person. So this doesn't mean that Cushing's or *bilateral adrenalectomy* (BLA) will cause these, but for me it exaggerated my issues to the strongest degree.

I can honestly say now that I was—and had been—addicted to food. I used food to calm my anxiety and soothe and numb my pain. Eventually the pain I felt from overeating replaced the pain I felt elsewhere. This pain now became what I craved, my new normal, and without it my anxiety would grow. All of these things, of course, are all the wrong reasons one should use food, and is considered an unhealthy relationship with it. Food is supposed to be for fuel...not comfort, not celebration. But life is more fun that way. I get it. But sometimes certain food affects your immune system, brain function, and your daily life. Living happy and healthy daily should be more important than the few minutes of enjoyment we get from bad food. I sometimes say, "Food almost killed me." It really did. I was a shell of a person dying inside with no mental capacity to cope with stress.

When I tried to diet, the hunger pains and headaches were so severe that I would oftentimes come home from work and take a sleeping pill just so I would not have to feel the discomfort. I ate way more than I truly needed, and because Cushing's is a metabolic disease, the body no longer knows what to do with sugars, proteins and fat. Therefore it stores it, usually in your midsection and base of the neck to protect your vital organs.

The effects of cortisol overload on the body aside, food is medicine and you are what you eat. I fought this fact for years, hoping I could feel better without changing my diet. I had always eaten pretty healthy but I also enjoyed my life and splurged often. They say most trainers do everything to the extreme, we work hard, play hard, and party harder. This was especially true when the possible MS diagnosis came about and I was lost, running around town to doctors, leaving each appointment crying after each neurologist or endocrinologist would say, "I'm sorry, in all my years, I have never seen an attack like this. I'm sorry I can't help." So I'd make my way to McDonald's for my drug of choice: BigMac, fries and an M&M McFlurry. Yep, I was a true addict. The eating disorders and body image issues most personal trainers have can become severe. I was in a downward spiral that I couldn't get out of.

The reactions I felt, like walking around drunk at times, so lethargic and out of it. Each hour I would be looking for some type of food to give me a boost of energy, or make me feel better.

One day I was driving through the city, having a huge pity party for myself as I watched people standing outside McDonald's eating a huge meal. I was jealous, thinking why could others eat whatever they wanted and be skinny and have the energy to spend time with their families but I couldn't? I was jealous of the women with strollers having coffee together. How did they have energy to raise a child and still meet up with their friends? Pity parties are okay once in a while but I'm sure if I talked to that person, I would realize they, too, are dealing with struggles I could never imagine. Kind of puts it all in perspective. I tried to put a positive spin on it, sometimes thinking, okay I'm dealing with so many health issues that that means God will not also make me deal with other tragedies in life such as the death of a family member or other crisis because he knows just how much we can handle. I looked at it like a positive, as if my health issues would shield me from another tragedy.

I often wondered why I was so stubborn. Why did I have to get to the bottom of the barrel to try to make a change? Why couldn't I just realize early on that I had to make healthy choices, and that meant even stricter choices than the average person. They say God places challenges in your way to help you grow and change. That the severity of the change represents the crux of your wellbeing. I finally started to get it...guess I'm a slow learner.

I hated waking up every morning with the all-intrusive thought of what I was going to eat that day, my brain spinning with: would I get a stomach ache, would it tide me over until I got to eat again, would I want to kill everyone around me because I didn't make it back to the house in time—or would I just give up and promise to start eating better tomorrow, pull through a quick drive thru, spending the rest of the night shaming myself because I wasn't strong enough to fight it. I exhausted myself.

For some reason I was always hungry, never feeling full and satisfied. They say 80% of personal trainers have some form of body image issue or eating disorder. I would have to agree. When you spend your life in hyper-touch with how you look, it plays tricks on your mind and you often set unrealistic body type goals for yourself.

I try to look at it now as if to compare to my friend Candy, who cuts, colors and styles hair. She is a perfectionist, so if she does someone's hair, while it may look wonderful and perfect to me, a real stylist like her would see all the flaws. How certain areas of the hair didn't lay as planned, the tone and color were slightly off. These are things I would never see as a regular person. I hope the same applies to personal trainers. We look at our bodies and notice every dimple and curve but to the everyday person we look great!

For me, if I were to add up all the hours spent researching diets, talking about diets, thinking about what I wanted to change in my diet, and obsessing over my health, I would have to take years off my life. If we used only one-quarter of the energy spent thinking, talking, obsessing about our health and actually put it toward taking the actual steps needed to put those thoughts into play, we would be golden. Remember, there is no magic pill—if there was, I'd have found it by now! However, there might just be a magic hormone!

Leptin, the "Satiety" Hormone

A client once asked me if I'd heard about the hormone leptin. I had not, so one day while waiting for my husband, I turned to a podcast on my iPhone. I saw leptin in one of the titles—I clicked on it, just killing time. I was fascinated, learning that it is the hormone released to feel "satiated or satisfied" and oftentimes people are leptin-resistant, similar to insulin resistance.

For example, have you ever eaten a meal and then wanted more, and then even more, and all of a sudden you were over-stuffed and full? This is because of a delay in your brain receiving the signal from leptin letting you know to stop eating. Had you gotten the signal earlier, you would not have continued to eat, but felt satisfied. This started making total sense to me.

I was always hungry, I rarely felt satisfied until I was so stuffed that I was in physical pain. I tried to piece it together. In my opinion, if Cushing's causes your body to think *fight or flight* crisis mode, then it's always going to get a signal that I need more energy, I need more food. If we can calm that anxiety and constant desire to need something (I calmed it with food, others calm it with alcohol, drugs, etc.), then we can decrease our cortisol, decrease stress in the body, and allow the body to heal!

I wanted to learn more about leptin so I attended a five-day retreat that taught you all about it, including how to prepare food correctly. It was eye-opening! I never thought it was possible to eat such decadent food and still lose weight. It recommended the fastest way to improve leptin resistance is a diet high in good fats, such as avocado, coconut oil, etc., and low in carbs and moderate protein. This went against everything I ever learned as a personal trainer. We were all about no fat, high protein. And wait, no sugar? I would not have believed it if I had not experienced it for myself.

Now I know there is not a person out there who says "Yay! I have to give up sugar! I couldn't be more excited!" Believe me, I have tried everything to get around it.

Depending on your body type, you would choose to stay below either 50-60 grams of carbs per day, or if you are strict keto you would stay under 20 grams of carbs per day. However, if you choose to do high fat, you *must* keep your carbs low. You cannot bounce back and forth between high fat-low carb, then go crazy on the weekends.

When I go above my allowance of carbs for a few days, my cravings and odd hunger headaches return, that anxious feeling in my stomach of needing something but I can't figure out what, returns and my irritability and motivation is noticeably altered.

As I said earlier, I truly feel I was addicted to food. I wish I could come up with a workout or pill that allows you to eat whatever you want and still lose weight and be healthy. Believe me, we've all tried, but we know it doesn't exist. But a high fat-low carb diet seemed to work best for my brain, mood, and energy level. I was feeling great and was only using food as my medicine, not to numb or escape! Could this be, could food alone have this much impact on my health. The answer is *absolutely*!

Ketosis

Over the next few weeks I had more energy and felt more alive than I had in my entire life! Oh, and I happened to lose over 20lbs the first month! I had no headaches, neck muscular tension, brain fog, dark thoughts or depression or anxiety, sugar cravings, my blood sugar stabilized, and no hunger. Of course I'd say *yes* to anything that can help with even one of those symptoms.

I went on an energy-filled spree, organizing and cleaning top-to-bottom my entire house, cabinets and junk drawer, silverware drawers, pots and pans and even my clothes closets. Each day was a new beginning and I was excited to take on the world. This was a new life and new beginning for me. The key to my personal success was a combination of stabilizing my dosing of steroid, hormones and anxiety/depression medication, doing a "leaky gut cleanse," followed by a ketogenic diet with intermittent fasting. (See my "Top 10 things I did to succeed" chapter.)

My husband saw me change before his eyes. He started calling me "superwife." He wanted to feel the same, so three weeks before his birthday he decided to give ketogenics (remember no fruit, sugar, gluten, etc) a try. One Sunday morning I woke up and found a small grape stem on the counter. "TIM," I yelled. "Did you eat a grape?" He stared at me like a deer in the headlights, hung his head in defeat and said "YES, I ate some grapes, I couldn't take it anymore. It was Saturday night I was just sitting here drinking water. I don't know how you do it!" I expressed my disappointment as he walked back upstairs. "Man, Shi, you'd think you found some cigarettes and dollar bills, but no, I get busted for a grape stem." Now that's funny!

Well, he made it through the weeks leading up to his birthday, lost 13 lbs and felt the healthiest he has in years with a little added sympathy for me. Not bad.

How Ketosis Works

Your body basically goes on two sources of energy. Either you are a glucose burner or a fat burner. Most of us are glucose burners, simple carbs and sugars are readily available for our energy source. However, we burn through them very quickly, meaning we also need to replenish them often. As a personal trainer, we are taught to eat every two-and-a-half to three hours to keep our fuel burning. However, this is a challenge when you also have to restrict your calories. In order to tap into your fat stores there must be a *deficit* of calories-in versus calories-out (I always hated that phrase but now it's making more sense to me the more I learn). And as we know, all calories are not created equal.

The other energy source the body can run off of is fat, and this is also what our brain functions best on. It's a slow-burning, long-sustainable energy. During the first week of ketosis you are basically cutting off your body's energy source by taking away the sugar and carbs. Your body freaks out because it doesn't know what to do. This is called the *keto flu*—eventually your body adjusts and then understands that you now want to use fat as its energy source, thereby kicking into a different energy source—*fat*—and you become a fat burner.

When in ketosis, you are able to use food for what it was meant for...fuel. You don't feel a "low blood sugar, give me anything at all because I'm starving" sensation, but rather you notice the brain's normal signal, a little feeling in your stomach, when it's time to eat. You can enjoy decadent, rich food that fills you up quickly and you're off to live the rest of your life. Some people choose to stay under 50grams of carbs per day, while the best benefits are gained when you stay under 20grams per day.

Along with the amazing surge of energy, there's a decrease in hunger because your brain is getting the signal, "Ah okay you want me to burn fat, well I have plenty of that." It is no longer in crisis mode. You start going longer and longer with high energy (and not from sugar-laden energy drinks that are horrible for you) and no intense desire for food at all times. This is because you don't experience the blood sugar drop and mood swings every "Cushie" knows all too well. I always thought this would be especially beneficial for nurses or anyone who goes long hours without being able to eat. You do not experience the sugar crash all of a sudden when someone needs you. Your stomach simply starts to feel a little hungry and you get to eating when you're ready. No more "hungry grocery shopping trips" we are all guilty of. The brain is now getting the message you are no longer in crisis mode, so it can stop throwing out cortisol and you can calm down because we have plenty of energy source in fat!

Yet a little bit more about **ketogenic:** Honestly, 90% of my daily symptoms went away when I switched to a ketogenic diet. No crazy hunger pains or sugar cravings, no headaches, migraines, neck pain, nausea, depression, anxiety. My skin is glowing, my cheek bones returned, I noticed I don't cough up phlegm in the morning like I did my entire life, I no longer get acid reflux and heartburn, all totally gone! Mentally, I feel like I finally have a sharp mind, always remembering what I have to do next. I don't get overwhelmed easily, my stomach is definitely flatter now that I have no inflammation from gluten, and no random stomach pains from being bloated or sudden cramping. I can see my muscles more, and my sight is clear. A nice side-effect of this is I'm actually saving money by eating organic because I only eat a few times a day. For me, one of the most important things is I am focusing on the rest of the joys of my life not being tormented by food.

It's important to say that I do question whether the body sees ketosis itself as a *stress*, thereby causing problems. I have tried to research this diligently online but it seems as if every doctor talking about it is looking through their own specialty, and health fanatics don't seem to have—or have had—the unique symptoms we are dealing with. I also wonder if ketosis affects pituitary or ectopic Cushing's patients differently than adrenal. Either way, no one can argue that getting rid of gluten, processed foods, and sugar is bad for you. Ketosis is not for everyone, and depends on certain factors in your life. If your cortisol or hormones are not stable, you will have a harder time with it. Anyone breast feeding or with some thyroid conditions should talk to their doctor first before doing any of these large dietary changes. Make sure to stay tuned to my website, listed in the covering pages, for more info as I continue to explore this topic. And I cannot stress this part enough: **always check with your doctor first!**

Reviews and Suggestions on Diet and Cleanses*

I would like to start this section by saying that I am simply giving my reviews and experiences on diets, cleanses, and fasts I've tried. I am not endorsing or receiving reimbursement for any of the items I talk about. Remember that "diet" means a *way of eating*.

Colorado Cleanse (14 days): This was the first cleanse my brother Michael talked me into before I was diagnosed. It uses a combination of Ayurvedic herbs, healthy eating, meditation, yoga, and a reset for your digestive tract. It goes in three phases: The first prepares your liver to be able to filter all the toxins that are going to be released. This is a crucial part of any cleanse, and without it the liver can possibly recirculate toxins throughout body and brain. The second provides you with seven days of a mixture of basmati rice and mung bean with Indian herbs and ghee, that is a complete meal and easy on the digestive tract. The third prepares you to go back to normal eating by re-introducing certain foods back into your diet. This cleanse was done when I was full Cushing's, although I do feel the herbs interfered with my blood work (so I do not recommend this if you are currently testing). This was my first attempt at a cleanse and I felt *amazing*! I had a blood analysis done before and after, and it literally changed and cleaned my blood. The side-by-side comparison of the blood was an amazing motivator. I personally recommend this cleanse to anyone. It is very detailed, though, and can be overwhelming. My first time, I just chose certain parts I wanted to focus on and slowly added in the rest once I got the rhythm down. I went on to have over 30 friends, family, and clients complete it. I have the routine down pat, so reach out if you're interested, I can definitely help you through it.

Leaky Gut Cleanse, or liver prep: Before starting any diet or cleanse, I recommend a "leaky gut cleanse" or liver prep first. The first resets the good flora and bacteria in your digestive tract by focusing on probiotic and fermented foods such as sauerkraut, kimchi, and kefir, along with nutrient-rich organic bone broth. It heals the walls of your intestines in order to absorb the already lacking nutrients of the good food we do eat.

The liver prep focuses on beets and a lot of green vegetables such as celery, zucchini, green beans, and the herb parsley. All are wonderful for prepping the liver to be ready for what's to come.

By the way, I paid $500 for a 30-minute Skype call to a doctor in California, who suggested doing these steps before any cleanse, diet or ketogenic diet. Although it hurt to pay, I can truly say it was a game-changer. He explained that steroids, NSAIDS, antidepressants, birth control, etc., wreak havoc on your digestive tract and stomach. Some days I was taking as many as 25-31 pills just to get through. My system was shot and not able to recover from even the smallest thing. The leaky gut cleanse healed my digestive tract and allowed me greater benefits of any diet.

Strict Low Carb: I also tried an extreme form of high fat, very low carb diet. It was more for people dealing with extreme health issues such as seizures, and promotes as little carbs as possible. However, unlike the Colorado Cleanse, it allows alcohol-free Stevia sweetener and several options for a sweet tooth, which I liked. Again, I felt amazing but often felt it was a little too strict to maintain with extremely low carbs. A good balance is always key.

Whole 30, Paleo: There is also the "Whole 30" or "Paleo" diet. Both are clean eating and allow complex carbs such as sweet potato, and minimal fruit such as berries. For most, this is the diet that works best. However, for me, for some reason even the slightest bit of carbs, even good carbs, makes me crave more and more. Like any good addict, I can't have just one. As I mentioned earlier, the only way to tap into your fat stores is if there is a deficit, which equals hunger and cravings. I cannot make good healthy decisions when I am hungry. Therefore, this is not my recommended diet method.

Low carb-high fat ketogenic, strict ketogenic: A ketogenic diet (which causes the body to be in *ketosis*) is obviously what worked best for me. It's nice because you still feel like you are cheating if you go out to dinner and have a periodic splurge on chicken wings and blue cheese. Or a cheeseburger wrapped in lettuce. Or even pork rinds (yes, I said pork rinds since they have no carbs or sugar) dipped in spinach artichoke dip. This is only an occasional thing, but if you were a sugar burner, then you would not be able to even think about this splurge without guilt. Overall, the increased energy, along with decreased hunger, cravings, less inflammation, less random aches and pains, stabilized blood sugar, and no brain fog makes this my new lifestyle. I know this diet is highly debated, but honestly you could not pay me to go back to how bad I felt before when not staying in ketosis.

Intermittent fasting: After you gain the benefits of ketosis and lose the weight you want, you will be hooked. The next level is to move onto intermittent fasting. Once in ketosis, you are not hungry anyway and have tons of energy. The intermittent fast is a way of giving your digestive tract a break so it can heal other things by simply skipping breakfast, and is usually a 16-hour fast. For example, let's say breakfast is 8am, lunch 12pm, and dinner 8pm—simply go from 8pm dinner until lunch the next day to complete a 16 hour-fast. I had no problem doing this after several weeks in ketosis.

Other fasts: I tried some things just to experiment so that I could share what happened, good and bad. The doctors were so unfamiliar with how food affects each disease. I was willing to use my body as an experiment so I could share with you all the effects. However, I do *not* recommend going any further than a 16-hour fast if you are in ketosis. I have tested a three-day organic bone broth cleanse, and a seven-day bone broth, bentonite clay and psyllium husk cleanse. Done correctly, I have never felt better in my entire life. For some reason, my digestive tract takes so much of my energy. The least work I had to do, the more energy could be spent on healing the rest of me.

Suggestions no matter what plan you choose:

If you want to start eating healthy, make a plan to go grocery shopping on a Sunday, have a list with you to use to cook a few meals ahead that day. Get healthy snacks to have on hand so you are prepared for last minute changes. Schedule another time a few days later to cook a few more meals. Keep a small and large cooler bag and ice packs ready to bring your food everywhere with you. You must stay focused and prepared to succeed. Once you've made the decision, you'll find it's not daunting, and even really enjoyable to experiment with healthy versions of the foods you've always loved!

Food Tips

I now look at food totally differently—I get excited to put more and better stuff in my body, having learned to tell the difference between thirst and hunger, anxiousness and hunger. I would picture the damage that the bad food would do to me inside...negative imagery seemed to work well.

But now, I was in control, feeling what each healthy meal was doing to me to move me towards feeling better and better. Whenever I started feeling out of control of what was going on in my body, it gave me a sense of relief that I could control what was going *into* my body. I had had to reach rock bottom, though, to finally submit to the process and accept that I would never be one of those people who could eat whatever and get away with it. After I started using food for my benefit, it started paying off.

Through all of the above, 95% of my symptoms went away even post-surgery and post-Cushing's. I have lost 40lbs and am back to where I was before I got sick.

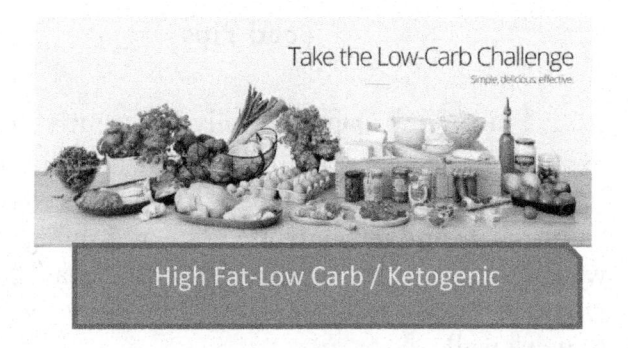

Take the Low-Carb Challenge
Simple, delicious, effective.

High Fat-Low Carb / Ketogenic

*Disclaimer: Before starting any new diet, cleanse, or exercise program, please check with your doctor and clear any exercise and/or diet changes with them before beginning. I am NOT a doctor, nutritionist or registered dietitian.

New-Found Youth at 40!

This year I celebrated my 40th birthday. Since Yosemite National Park is my favorite place on earth, I wanted to wake up that morning in the valley of Yosemite and hike Yosemite Falls Trail. My supportive husband, along with my best friend from San Francisco, Nina, joined me on this birthday quest, making it one of the most special and memorable times of my life. I'm a lucky woman.

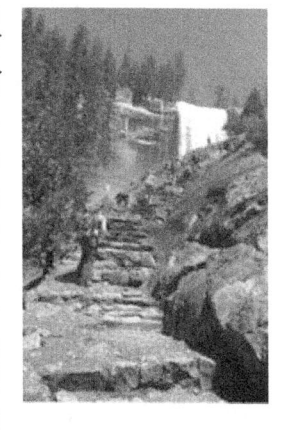

I took all the necessary precautions, up-dosing (correctly!) prior to the hike, having extra medication on me, as well as my emergency Solu-Cortef injection if needed (think of it like always having an epi-pen if you're allergic to peanuts or bees). It was a beautiful day out, perfect weather, and because the snowfalls had been record-breaking, the waterfalls were at the best they had ever been. Prior to us going to Yosemite, my husband dedicated two songs to me: *Fight Song* and *Even If We Can't Find Heaven, I'll Walk Through Hell With You*. I can't begin to describe how much this meant to me...he indeed had walked through hell with me, even though when we got married I promised him heaven. He stood by me, always believing in me, sometimes more than I believed in myself. I have those two songs on my iPod and at one particular time in the hike, the terrain was flat—with those songs playing on my iPod, a burst of energy surged through me and I took off running. I hadn't run in years! With the music filling all of me, I breathed deeply of the fresh mountain air. I grabbed my phone to capture the moment on video (it's posted on my website). We did the hike in seven hours, becoming one of my greatest accomplishments considering all I had been through.

With my health finally in order and feeling amazing, it was time to *"get Shi back"*...this meant to get back all the things this disease had taken from me, and getting back everything that made me *me:* My love for nature, exploring new things, traveling, physical effort that I so enjoyed even if it was at my "new norm," actually being in the moment and enjoying it with my loved ones without negative intrusive thoughts, music that motivated me instead of closing my eyes and using it to escape my world. This time my eyes were wide open. This was the moment when I knew I had made it through to the other side!

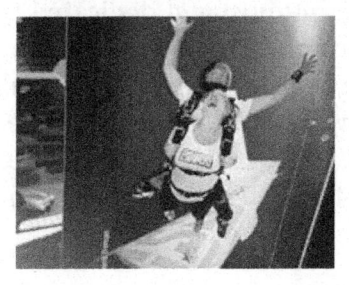

Skydiving in Dubai

BE YOUR OWN DOCTOR

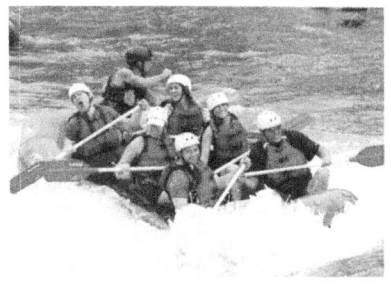

Whitewater rafting

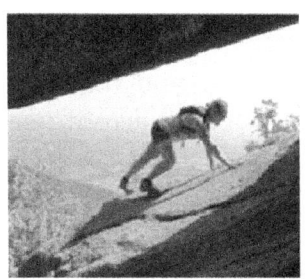

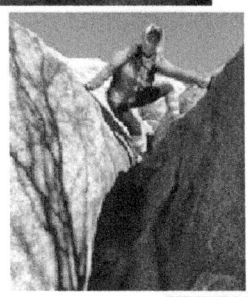

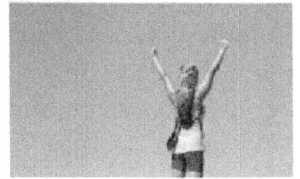

TRIUMPH!

Top 10 Things I Did To Succeed

Here are the top 10 things I focused on to "get my life together":

1: **Lower Cortisol.** First you must identify the source of high cortisol and stabilize it through medication, radiation, or pituitary or adrenal surgery.

2: **Proper Dosing.** Adjust and find a stable dosing schedule of Cortef and Fludro (if needed) with your Endocrinologist.

3: **Primary Care Physician.** A well-versed doctor to pull it all together.

4: **Medication and Hormones.** Address any chemical and/or hormonal imbalances from anxiety or depression from your psychiatrist. Stabilize or address hormonal imbalances with your gynecologist.

5: **Therapist and Support Group.** Find a professional psychologist to talk through your struggles. Find people online who are going through what you are and can relate. Sometimes you will need to just vent to someone who understands.

7: **Focus Outward.** When things get really tough for you, sometimes it's best to give your mind a break from obsessing over your health and *help someone else*. It makes you feel in control of something and positive. I love the saying, "If something good is not happening to you, maybe you're the good thing that's supposed to happen to others."

8: **Sleep.** Ensure you are sleeping enough and with quality. Get a sleep study for sleep apnea and possible needed CPAP.

9. ***Physical Therapist / Personal Trainer / Nutritionist.*** Some insurance companies cover physical therapy. Use this to start with: getting out of the house and doing monitored movement (have someone with you) so you do not injure yourself. Finding health care professionals familiar with Cushing's is a challenge, but if you find one willing to learn and go through it with you, that's golden. If not, reach out to me online. I can do Skype personal training and programs. Most importantly, clean up your diet, whatever that means for you. Take everything in baby steps, maybe just pick two things each week you're going to change. But overall, find what eating plan works well for you. No gluten; no sugar; no processed foods; Paleo; vegan; Ketogenic, intermittent fasting.

10. ***Slow Down*:** Try to find your new normal. Allow yourself down time between doctor appointments. Each can be emotionally draining.

Concluding Thoughts

I wanted to take a moment to reflect on some takeaways through my journey...

I hate that my childhood was so stressful to me. But I love that I learned the work ethic I have.

I hate that my career made me focus on my body. My life was saved because my career made me focus on my body.

I hate that the doctors dropped the ball so many times. I love that they made me "Be my Own Doctor."

I hate that my worst fears came true. I love that I have none left.

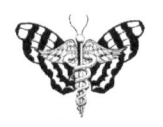

PART TWO

Exercises—From Hospital to Hikes

Now I know Cushing's is different for every person. The length of time and the damage done are sometimes hidden until put into use. But it's **never** too late to get strong!

When I got to the point I am today, I decided to dedicate my practice to, and specialize in, fitness for Cushing's survivors and anyone suffering from a chronic illness. So here are some fitness tips, starting with the easiest situation and leading you through the different levels. You can choose which applies to you.

As a side note, I'd like to announce here that I am developing a workbook for recording exercises and progress. A little motivational tool!

To start things off, when you are lying in the hospital during your recovery or if you are currently in a wheelchair prior to surgery, you can always have someone assist you in moving your joints if you cannot do it yourself. As a personal trainer I use PNF (proprio neuromuscular facilitation) stretching for my clients. This is where basically they lie on the floor or bed and I do most of the work. It is very nice if you can find a massage or physical therapist, or even a friend, who can move your legs, hips and joints in different directions for you.

If you are simply lying in bed, you can lift your own leg and bend your knees into your chest. Do this several times, lifting your leg as high as you can (it's okay if it's only a little at first) so the blood flow circulates back to the heart. There's a reason they place the "leg squeezers" on you to increase blood flow and decrease risk for blood clots.

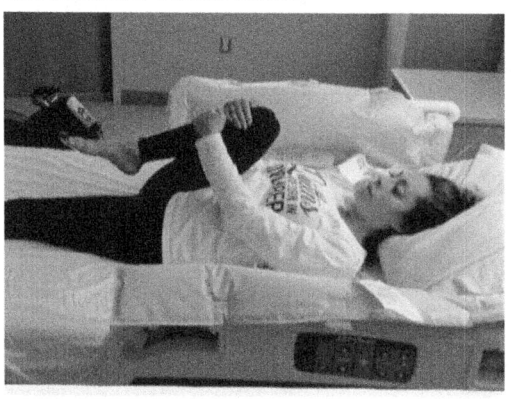

If you are lying down, sit up to the edge of your bed. Then slowly lower yourself back down to a lying position. Do this several times in a row. When we are going through our everyday life, we have to stop to realize that everything we do uses different muscle groups—so we are simply taking our everyday life and making it into a workout! Have a goal of 10 before you stop to take a break. If you can't at first, then just try, that's the *most important* thing. Work your way up to two or three sets of 10 of each movement.

Most people say they cannot do a squat. But you get out of bed every morning right? A good one for starters is to simply stand up off of the bed. You can use your hands to push off the bed into a standing position, then **slowly** lower yourself back down to sit on the edge of your bed holding your abdominals in. Do this several times in a row, counting to see how many you can do without discomfort. Even if it's one or two to start, you are moving! Do this every day a couple times and slowly you will find yourself doing three, four, even ten.

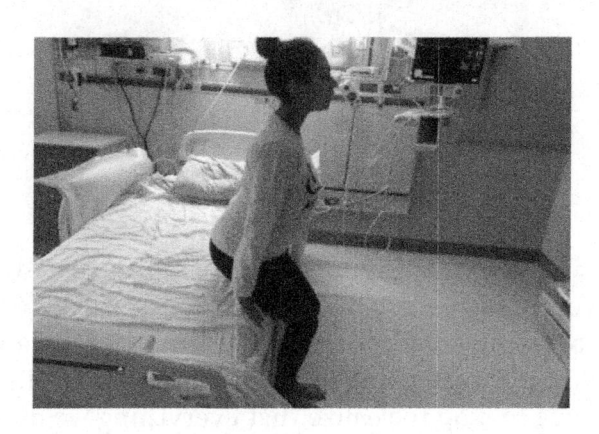

Doing wall push-ups is great for stretching and using the arm muscles. Put your hands on the wall in front of you, walk your feet back, choosing an angle that allows you to touch your nose to the wall. Then push yourself back as if you were doing a push-up on the ground. This is considered a modified push-up, and the stretch feels great in your arms.

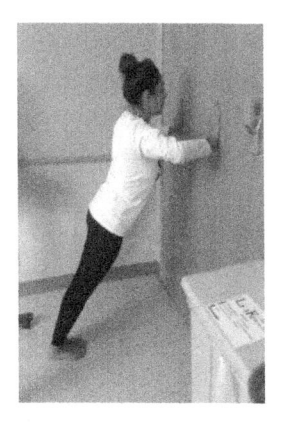

For some core work, modify a plank by placing your elbows on a counter. Walk your feet back slowly and hold this position. You are now strengthening your mid-section muscle group, abs, side obliques, and low back!

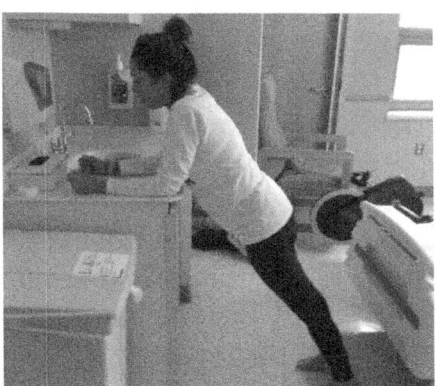

For this next one, a row for the back, I recommend getting a small resistance band, simply tying it around a banister or your feet.

You can do this from a seated or standing position. Squeeze your shoulder blades together, without shrugging your shoulders. This is great for releasing that stress that our body carries in the shoulders and neck. That's why a massage feels so good. This is an excellent one for those of us who are behind a computer often, answering emails and stressful phone calls. But the problem is we aren't moving the body to release that stress, so it just stays there getting more and more tense, building in our neck and shoulders. Squeeze your shoulder blades together first, then pull back with the arms. Do this as many times as you can and record your progress.

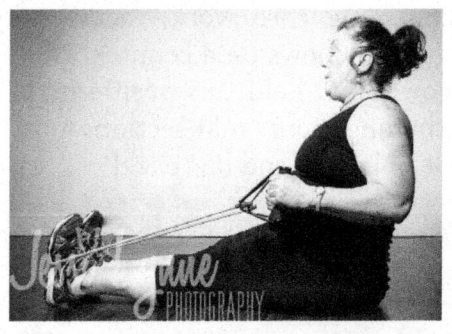

Another good exercise is to simply lie on the floor with your knees bent. Tuck your hips and attempt to press the small of your lower back against the floor. See the natural curve in the low back of the first photo. Then flatten back like in second photo. Hold this position for 5-10 seconds. You can add an upper body lift when you are ready, lifting several times (this is called a modified crunch).

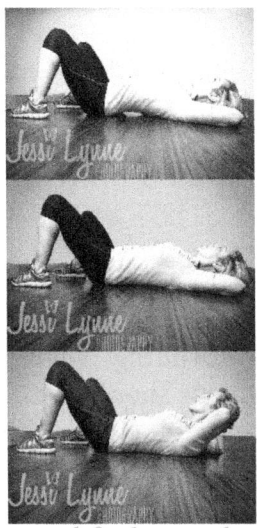

Modified Crunch

A physical therapy exercise used often for those recovering from back surgery is called *the bridge.* Lie on your back on the floor, pressing your heels into the floor and lifting your hips up as high as you can, even if only a few inches, squeezing your glutes (buttock muscles). Keep your upper back and shoulders on the floor. Return to rest position. Do this as many times as comfortable and record. Again, try to increase by two more each time. This exercise works the entire back chain of the body, the low back, gluteal, and hamstrings. It's one of my own personal favorites to do.

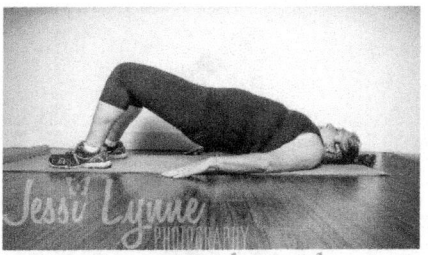

The Bridge

The *modified plank* involves lying on your stomach and bending your knees with your elbows under your shoulders. Lift your hips up off the floor, while doing something called a pelvic tilt. This is similar to what you did when you were lying on your back and you placed your low back against the floor. You will hold this plank on your knees and time yourself for how many seconds you can hold it. Each day try to beat the number from the day before. (**Note:** *Photo 1 is modified plank set WRONG with arched back and head up—Photo 2 is the modified plank set CORRECTLY.*)

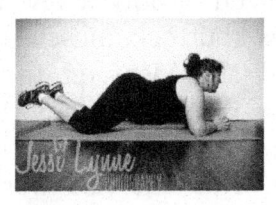

Wrong body placement

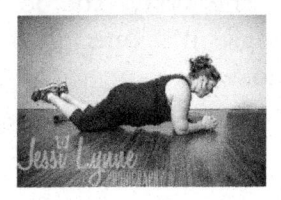

Right body placement

Swimming is always a great way to get moving, as it uses water for resistance. Using water weights or even simply moving your legs in the water as if you were doing various exercises, or swaying your body forward and back, or dancing, or doggie-paddling, or walking using the resistance of the water—they are all a fantastic, low-impact way to get lots of exercise and move, move, move—Soon you'll be doing water aerobics!

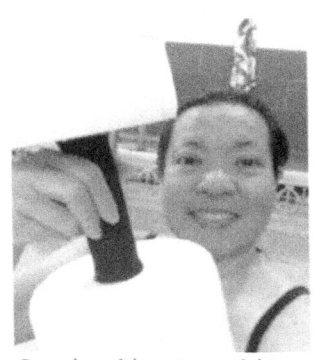

Brenda, with water weights

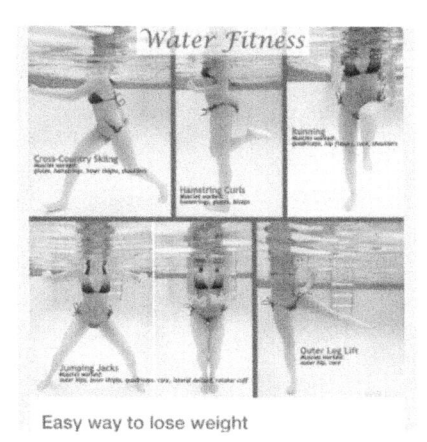

Easy way to lose weight

Dancing: No, you don't need to get up and dressed up and go out to some dance club...put on some music while you're housecleaning, or cooking, or even while sitting at the computer (if you do computer work or desk work at home). Just make sure you move, even if just a little bit!

Move, move, move...

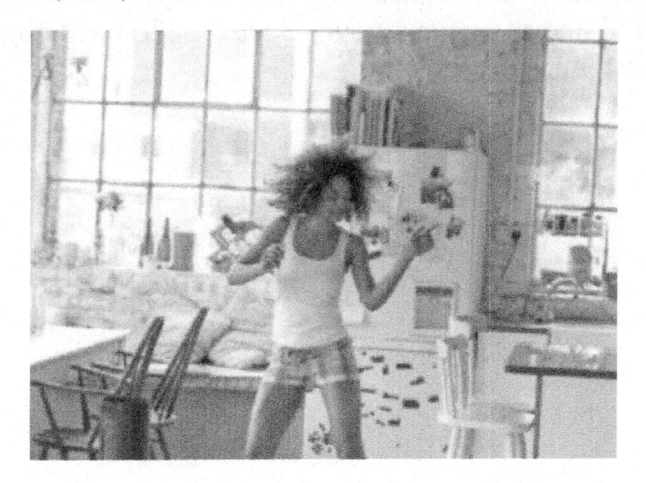

...like nobody is watching!

Stretches

Often in our everyday life we suddenly reach to grab something from a shelf or move in an awkward way to grab something out of a closet, behind a box, and in the corner. We must attempt to do these moves slowly, in a controlled environment such as during our workout, so that in our everyday life it is not so foreign to the body. If we are normally inactive and then suddenly need to move in odd ways to get the Christmas decorations out of the closet for holidays, we risk our bodies tensing up, pulling a muscle or injuring a joint. Moving regularly will allow the body to protect itself when life comes flying at us!

Rotation: Sit in a chair and slowly rotate, reaching behind you as if getting something out of the back seat of your car. Hold each position for as long as comfortable on the right side and then the left side.

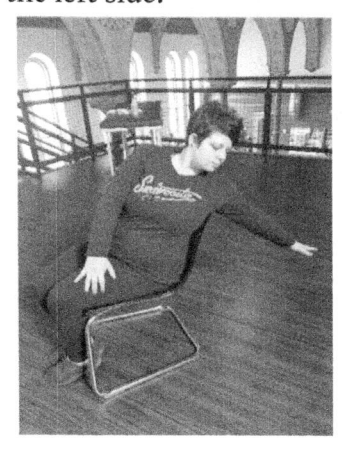

Side bend: Sit in a chair and very slowly bend to the side as if you're reaching to pick up a water bottle or pen off the floor. Do this repeatedly on one side. Record how many times you can do this without pain. If you are able to reach the floor successfully, the next step is to move the water bottle or pen slightly further away and try again.

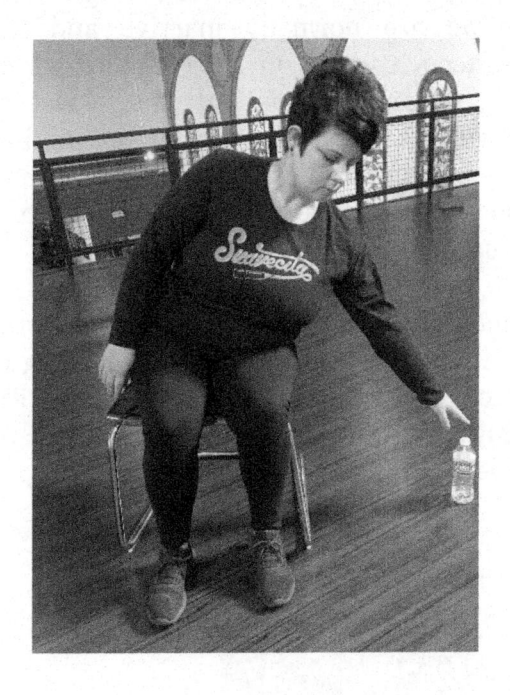

BASIC 6

For more advanced clients, I have what I call my **Basic 6.** These are the six basic movements that everyone should do when they go to the gym. We are often overwhelmed with all of the magazine articles and our friends influencing us on what exercises work the best. However, there are *motions* that incorporate several muscle groups at the same time, therefore maximizing your time efficiency.

#1 -- PUSH: The first exercise is a pushing motion. This can be a push-up on the wall, a push up on the ground on your knees/toes, or using the resistance band to do a chest press. You can change up the angles by doing an incline press, a straight ahead press, or an overhead press.

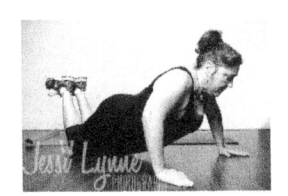

#2 -- PULL: Using the resistance bands, pull your shoulder blades together without shrugging your shoulders, like mentioned earlier. Pull the bands back as far as you comfortably can and repeat.

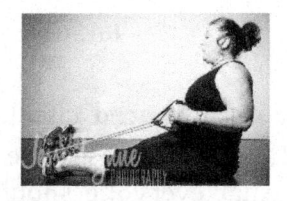

#3 -- PRESS: This refers to a leg press or standing squat, whichever your knees and hips can handle. Make sure your weight is back with pressure through your heels to protect the knees. Pull your abs in, shoulders back, and ensure good posture. This can be from standing up from your bed and slowly lowering yourself back down, to a squat with a bench behind you, or a leg press machine at the gym.

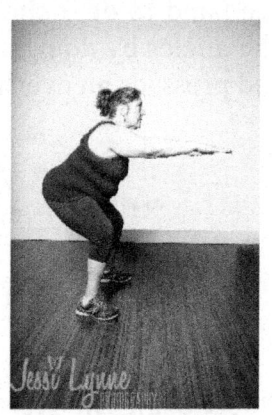

#4 -- BALANCE: Add a little balance exercise between each set. Standing on one leg, start to bring one heel off of the floor. Slowly lift your toe and hook your foot behind you. If you want to

further challenge yourself, lift your knee fully in the air.

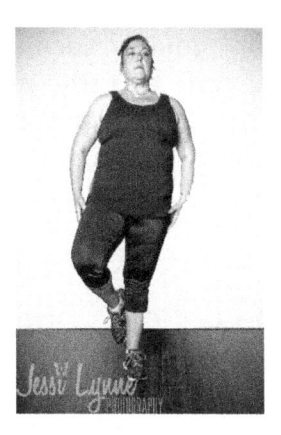

#5 -- CORE: I am personally a big fan of any modified plank that you can do. If not, you can simply lay flat on the floor and do the pelvic tilt as mentioned earlier. If you're ready to move on, plank on your toes for a greater challenge.

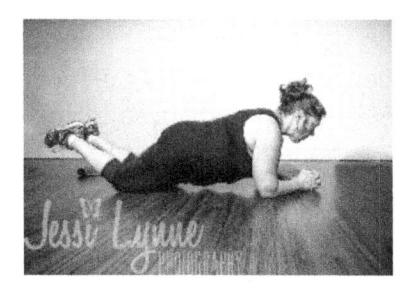

#6 -- CARDIO: Using the Polar® Heart Rate monitor, choose a speed and incline that is comfortable for you. You should be able to speak at least three words without taking a gasp for air. Take a look at your heart rate. See how long you can maintain that speed and intensity...five minutes, eight minutes? Each session attempt to increase your time by three minutes! (*Note*: the "wrist only" heart rate monitors are not nearly as accurate as the full chest strap Polar® heart rate monitors. I've tested them all.)

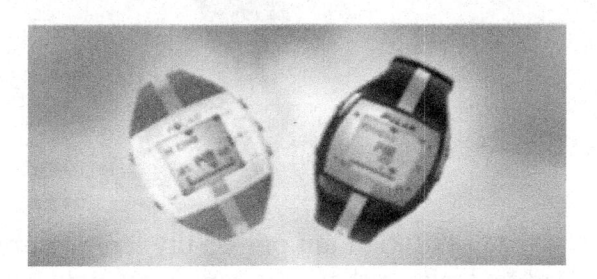

SUPER 3

When you are ready to move to the next level, I have combined three ultimate multi-joint (multiple joints moving at the same time) movements to hit every muscle in your body, challenge your balance, and increase your heart rate to include cardio, all in three amazing moves.

Push: Placing one foot forward and one foot back (this is called a split stance), bend the back knee towards the floor. As you straighten your legs, press your arms over your head.

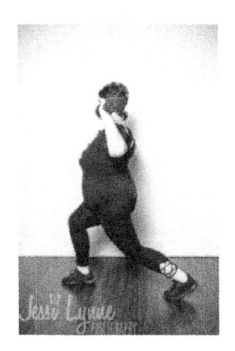

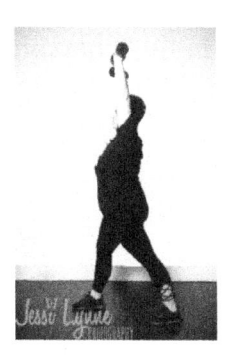

Pull: Place one foot forward and the other foot all the way back behind you. Keep the back leg straight and front knee bent. Hold this static deep lunge while doing a rowing motion with resistance bands.

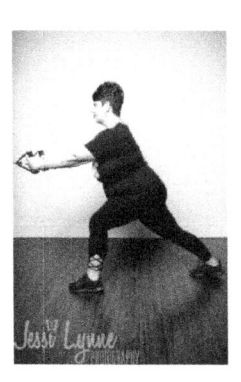

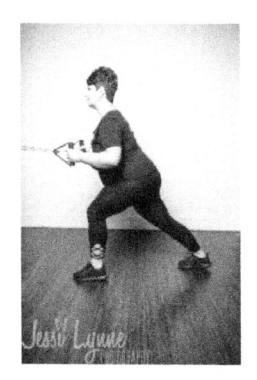

Rotation / Wood Chop: Bend your knees into a squat position. With arms straight, rotate only your upper body to one side (holding a small dumbbell for more of a challenge). Next, stand up and rotate the body to the opposite side in a low- to high- "chopping" motion.

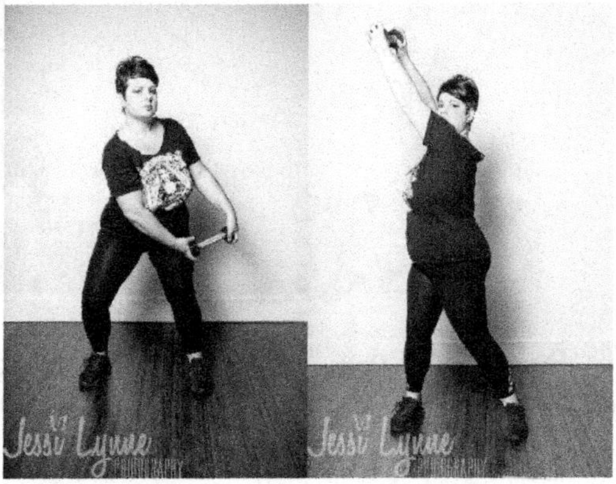

Photo L: Starting position, squat and rotate

Photo R: Ending position, stand and reach

Cushing's Beauty and Fashion Tips

We all know the horrific side effects of Cushing's: weight gain, muscle loss, hair loss, acne, skin rashes, facial hair, the stretch marks, just to name a few of the outer ones. Unfortunately, I am a very vain person and have always needed to keep up a certain image for my livelihood. Here are some things I did to manage the physical changes that were happening. Though I know that we are all beautiful no matter what, the changes our bodies go through with this disease can completely destroy any self-esteem we have. We know we can't control what's happening and that we can control our response—but we can't control how we are seen in society's eyes. It's not their fault necessarily, but it's the ignorance to this disease.

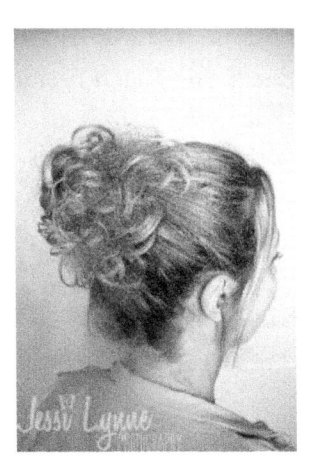

Hair loss: My hair was always my thing. When I went to the salon the stylist would always charge me extra because my hair was so thick. So as it started to thin, my friend Candy suggested getting extensions. I fought her on this for a while but she knew what was best. They were pretty expensive and I knew once I started I would want more. But looking back, her push truly helped me get through the hair loss and thinning. It was well worth it. For a less-expensive option, I also purchased a hairpiece from Ulta (I got the one called *curly bun*, though there are many others) for under $20. When I was going through hot flashes, heat intolerance and the summer months, I would pull my hair up in a bun and place this hairpiece over the bun. It looked like I just threw my hair up in a cute messy bun. It was amazing! I wish I had done both earlier.

For my *receding hairline*, I used *Style Edit Root Concealer*. I have a big forehead and long face to begin with, so it was nice to simply shade along the hair line and make everything look smaller. It's the little tricks that can help!

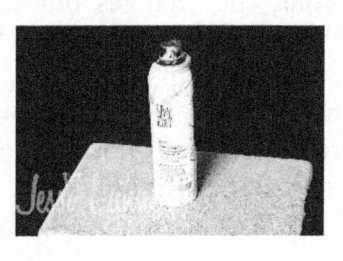

For *facial hair growth*, I used *One Touch Facial Trimmer*. It costs $10, and is easy to use. Sit in front of a window so the natural light can guide you. Some trimmers come with a mini-light that helps guide as well.

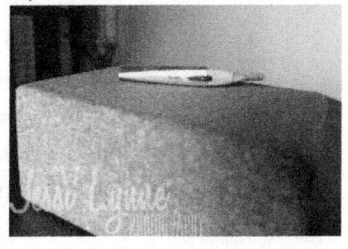

Moonface: Ah the ubiquitous rounding of the face called moonface! One of the most telling aspects of this disease, it was a constant reminder I was sick, every single time I passed a mirror. So I learned how to contour my cheekbones with bronzer. Taking it a step further, I included a highlighter and learned how to use it. It was an added bonus. I personally used *Bare Minerals-Warmth* and *NYX* contour kit.

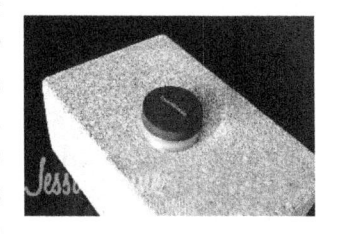

Weight gain: This is perhaps the hardest thing a "Cushie" has to deal with, and it can be unnerving, depressing and frustrating to adjust to weight gain and subsequent loss (post-surgical, and which has its own frustrations such as loose skin). Many times I would help my clients during the losing process learn how to shop for their body size. My new-found knowledge was, of course, due to having to learn how to shop for my own new larger size.

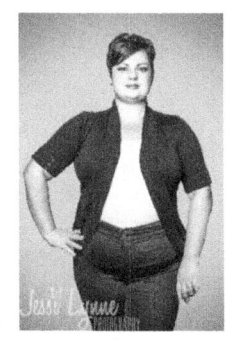

My first tip is black everything! To help with the self-esteem issues, it's a learning process to understand that, while we may not like it and always hear the negativity surrounding wearing black, we want to feel good about ourselves and

yes, it's okay to wear black! Focus on dark open sweaters with a light shirt. See how the lines of the sweater are very flattering.

Be careful to make sure your clothes are not too tight; for the females, be sure your bras fit correctly—ask at the shop, good stores will have knowledgeable salespeople to help with fit. A badly-fitted bra on women even without Cushing's will make a roll on the back. Invest in undergarments that smooth the skin and make you feel better. The US brand *Spanx* (also known as "spanks") is well worth the money! (In the pictures below, the bra and tank top are too tight. In the photo on the right, everything is smoothed out with the correct-sized shirt and undergarments.)

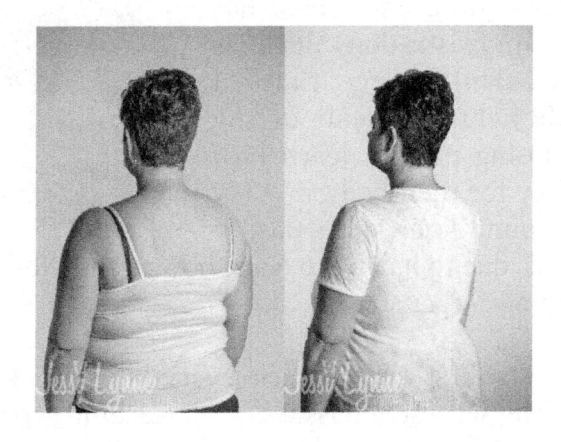

Invest in a pair of stretchy dark jeans. Don't forget all the many beautiful colorful scarves—not only do they add color, but they can help to cover the buffalo hump or fat deposit on the front neck, and mask the midsection.

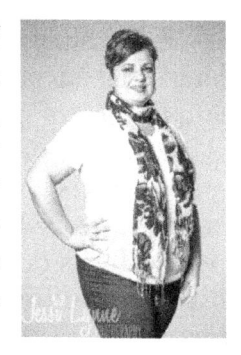

Cardigans were my best friend, but closed in front may look blocky. Try to keep them open, it essentially cuts you in half.

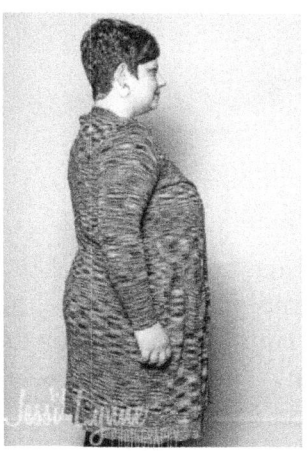

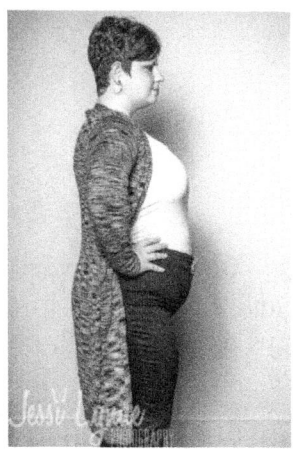

This is not a suggestion for everyone, because not everyone has an eyebrow (or facial hair) issue, but I did. So, I invested in getting my eyebrows permanently tattooed or *microblading*.

It was a birthday gift from my husband. With Cushing's, I had hair growth stop on the outer three-quarters of my eyebrows (many medical sites list this as a sign of adrenal fatigue and thyroid issues). The tattooed eyebrows (permanent brows) gave me something I could and would focus on while looking in a mirror, as opposed to scrutinizing every little thing on my *moonface*.

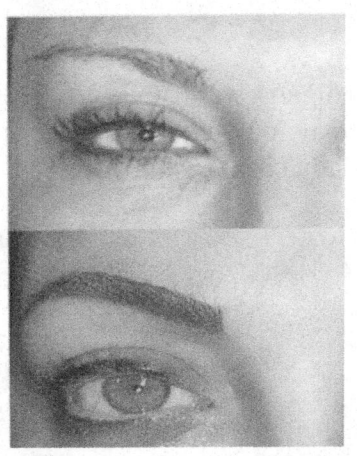

One of my favorite mascaras became *L'Oreal Double Extend*. It is in a red and white tube, and stays on really well, not running down your face like others can during our sweaty heat intolerance. You place first the white side on your lashes and then the black. It dries and can't be wiped off. The only way to take it off is with cleanser in a warm shower. It is quite an amazing product and stays on for days.

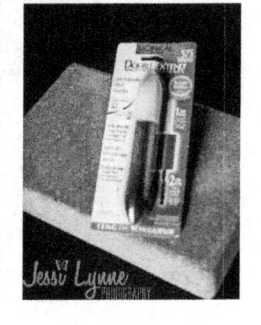

I used to like going to the nail salon, but of course with the rising medical bills, I couldn't afford it anymore. My friend, Lena, turned me on to *Kiss* nails, available at any drug store for about $7. They're a simple glue-on-and-press and come in length variations. I always got the *RS* for real short, and they were fantastic in the French manicure color. Just because we're wearing black in our clothes doesn't mean we can't also have dazzling and bright colors!

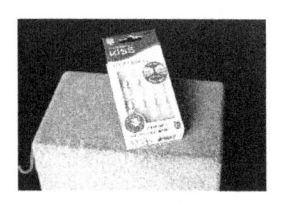

But a lot of this is really all about doing something completely different, new, something that excites us in this emotionally trying time—even a little thing like trying a new lipstick color. (I love *ColourPop Lipsticks*, which can only be ordered online for $8, and the colors last forever!) Trying a different style make up just gives you a little boost—and we all need all the help we can get *emotionally.*

Holistic and Alternative Therapy

On my quest for health, I was willing to try anything. Some worked, and some I did as an experiment just to be able to give an educated opinion. And now I can share some of these random things I tried with you!

Ayurvedic herbs: As I mentioned previously, I also attempted the *Colorado Cleanse* using Ayurvedic herbs. I probably had the best results with turmeric, manjistha, ashwagandha, black pepper, cinnamon (stabilizes blood sugar), and adaptogenic (natural substances thought to help the body adapt to stress) herbs. However, I have experimented with and without the herbs during bloodwork, and have found they **absolutely** affect your cortisol levels. So please make sure you are not on any supplements during crucial lab work.

One herb I particularly loved was called *gymnema* root. It's an interesting root that serves to "disengage" your brain's sugar taste buds[**] and ability to recognize sugar (it is periodically used for diabetics and food addicts to help decrease the desire for sugar). You open the capsule and place the contents on your tongue (tastes like cinnamon and bark), and sugary sweets will lose their taste. I have done this experiment on several clients—first having them taste some real sugar (tastes good), then placing the contents from the capsule on their tongue and giving them the same sugar. The response was that it tasted like *sand*. So if perhaps you're going to a party and know you will be tempted by sugary sweets, place the powder on your tongue and chances are you're not going to keep eating a cupcake that doesn't taste like anything! It's Ayurveda's best-kept secret. I don't know why I hadn't heard about this gem earlier in my career.

***Gymnema is **not** a long-term solution to sugar issues and shouldn't be used for more than 20 months continuously. It can affect blood sugar levels in people with diabetes (which is a common effect of Cushing's), so watch for the opposite signs of low blood sugar. Lastly, since it might have that effect, it can interfere with blood sugar control before and after surgical procedures. If you use it, then stop at least two weeks before any surgery. Of course, if you happen to be pregnant and/or breast feeding, don't take chances by using it. (WebMD, https://goo.gl/XppQ4Y)*

Acupuncture: I tried several different types of acupuncture as I believe in your Chi and energy. Because the high cortisol made me anxious, the Chi was high in my neck and head. I needed to redirect that energy down to my core and belly. Finding the right person with the right energy to apply the acupuncture is crucial as there are good and bad.

Coffee enema: Yes, I said coffee enema. My brother's wife had cancer and follows the Gerson method, which uses coffee enemas several times to detox the liver of all of the toxins that are being released. Needless to say, they are strong believers in it, and they convinced me to try it; it's now become a part of my regular health regimen. The caffeine in a coffee enema stimulates the liver to pump bile and clear the small duct that often gets clogged from poor nutrition, medications, and all the other toxins we eat and breathe. It's also useful if you have headaches or before/after vacation when you're not going to be able to eat (or haven't) as cleanly as you would like. There are several recipes on the web, but always remember to use organic ground coffee and distilled or filtered water, and mix in an enema bag. Lying on your left side, retain the fluids for 12-15 minutes. Just rest and breathe, as it can take some getting used to. Interestingly, during mine, I would lie on my side and just breathe and relax, *but* if I would reach for my phone when I remembered something work- or health-related, my internal muscles would contract and cramp. If I went back to relaxing and breathing normally, the internal cramping would go away. Minutes would go by, and I would reach for my phone if I heard a text—without fail, my internal muscles would contract and cramp, making it very painful. This felt so strange to me because I never would have felt this internal tension if I hadn't been in the middle of a coffee enema. It taught me just how sensitive our bodies are to stress and just how much its effects are subconscious, to the extent we don't realize what we are doing to our bodies.

Hydrocolonics: This is different from an at-home enema. Some spas offer hydrocolonics, which basically uses water pressure in and out to thoroughly cleanse the colon.

I also use a "Spotty Potty®" which is a foot stool you place at the base of your toilet. It places your knees slightly higher, positioning your body and colon for optimal elimination without straining.

Skin brushing for the ***lymphatic system*** is a good option to get your lymphatic system and energy moving, similar to Chi. It is an inexpensive brush you use before taking a shower, and then apply a lymphatic oil during the shower to get the system moving!

Chiropractics: I tested out several different practitioners, NUCCA, NAET, traditional, and I definitely believe in and highly recommend the benefits of a good chiropractor. Your spine is like a railroad track, with nerve endings feeding each organ a continuous blood supply—if the track is slightly off, the blood flow to that area is compromised. After 4-6 weeks with one type, if you aren't feeling relief, then don't continue wasting your time and money. Move on to a different technique or get scans to see if you are dealing with something structural.

Epsom salt baths: *Magnesium* is a cofactor in more than 300 enzyme systems that *regulate* diverse biochemical reactions in the body, including protein synthesis, muscle and nerve function, blood glucose control, and blood pressure regulation. Soaking in Epsom® salt is again one of my favorite things to do at night after an active day. It helps to relieve sore muscles and joint pain.

I also recommend switching to no chemicals, natural deodorant, and natural cleaning products, if possible. Milk of Magnesium® can be used as deodorant. Olivella® is my favorite all-natural, 100% extra virgin olive oil body wash. It's not oily and leaves your skin feeling really clean.

Massage: Do I even need to say the benefits and joy of massage?! Getting a massage every other week or at least once a month is highly recommended. It moves the lymphatic system, releases toxins and increases blood flow to areas you are not able to reach on your own. It relaxes your muscles, releases all the good endorphins, and it just feels amazing!

Sleep: Sleep is the most important thing you can do for your body. Remember, most of us had elevated cortisol levels even at night when the body needed to rest and repair, and so sleep became nearly non-existent it seemed. For years, I woke up with neck pain, headaches, and a crippling stiff back and hips. Invest in a good mattress and supportive pillow. Also, because our circadian rhythm is affected, it is important to go to bed and wake up at the same time as often as possible. I used natural sleep aides such as melatonin to help. Getting good rest is absolutely the best thing anyone, especially one with Cushing's, can focus on.

Please get a sleep study done even if it's before or after surgery. I was tested for sleep apnea, and it showed that unbelievably I stopped breathing 45 times per hour! I now sleep with a CPAP machine and am getting the true rest I needed for years. The mask takes some getting used to, but don't give up. Try different masks and head gear until you find a good fit. My husband uses a CPAP as well now. We joke that we are quite the couple going to bed at night, all geared up and wearing CPAPs with head gear—that includes a chin strap to hold your mouth closed, a bite plate for teeth grinding, ear plugs, eye mask, and a Fitbit to track sleep! Let me tell ya', we are SEXXY!!

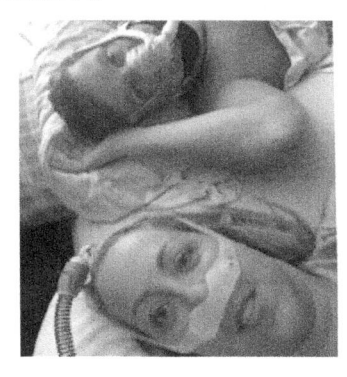

Supplements: I have been torn on this subject for years. I hate that supplements are not regulated and research studies show that only about 30% are actually what they say they are. However, I do believe our food is becoming more and more depleted of nutrients, so we need all the help we can get. I personally take fish oil, turmeric, holy basil, fiber, Vit D, Vit B and CBD oil. Follow my website as I further research reputable companies.

Water: We all know the supreme importance of getting enough fluids. It is one of the most important things you can focus on. I recommend trying for around 100 ounces per day. I get a sports bottle that's about 25 ounces and my goal is to finish two water bottles before noon, drink a third bottle before 3pm and the last before 6pm. This way it doesn't interfere with sleep and wake me up all the time to urinate! Try not to drink when eating meals, as it dilutes your digestive enzymes. Also, as hard as it was for me, I try to drink room temperature water verses ice cold. Part of the Colorado Cleanse I mentioned earlier, has you sip warm water throughout the day. It compares your digestive tract to a piece of leather. If you pour ice cold water on a piece of leather, it simply drips off. But if you slowly drip warm water on that leather throughout the day, it eventually softens; hence your digestive tract is better able to absorb the nutrients and water we take in! This fact became clear to me when my husband pointed out that on our six-hour car ride to Rochester, we only stopped once for me to use the restroom. He used to hate driving long distances with me because usually I would make him stop four or five times. We arrived at his mother's house, he smiled at me and said, "Now I *love* that cleanse, we only had to stop *once!*" It was amazing to me that something I resisted so much and was such a little change had made a world of difference.

Biofeedback: Breathing is everything and meditation is wonderful! Biofeedback is when you get hooked up to a machine that measures your heart rate, breath rate and/or brain activity. You complete exercises and attempt to slow your breathing to match the system on the screen. It accesses your parasympathetic nervous system. Oftentimes we are so stressed that we don't even realize we are holding our breath or breathing fast or doing short chest breathing rather than deep abdominal breathing.

Injections: I personally suffered from severe TMJ of the jaw, possibly from years of nervous habits of biting my lip or grinding my teeth when I sleep (I now use a bite plate when sleeping). The pain was daily and became unbearable. Someone suggested getting Botox in the mandibular joint. I thought that was crazy, spend money on Botox and not even get rid of wrinkles?! But I did some research and saw that it had worked for some. I did it and for me it was well worth it. The pain went away and I no longer needed ibuprofen...well at least not for that pain. Talk with your doctor or dentist before having it done.

A word about using cortisone creams and/or a one-time shot for something. I had had a nagging foot injury from about a year before surgery, called Turf Toe (basically I hyperextended my big toe). Sounds simple enough, but when every step is painful, you realize how much that big toe means to you. I went to a podiatrist who gave me a cortisone injection. I was scared to death because it was called *cortisone*. The one small shot provided enough anti-inflammatory for the toe to heal and I haven't had to get another since. I had a steroid injection for a bulging neck disk and while it dulled the pain about 30%, it didn't do much else and so wasn't worth it for me.

A question often asked by those pre- and post-Cushing's is whether cortisone topical creams for anti-inflammatory purposes or healing a cut, etc., are bad and will worsen or make your Cushing's return. Emphatically no! They are not going to "give you Cushing's" if you don't have it or are in recovery, or make your Cushing's worse. It is a different type of *cortisone*. You would probably need to spread the entire tube of cream on a piece of bread and eat it to have it affect you in that way.

Meditation: This was particularly challenging for me in the beginning. But like most, once you get it, you never know why you didn't try earlier. I don't recommend going to an hour long class like I did the first time. Just look up some YouTube videos and apps on your phone to guide you through. I try for about 15 minutes max, but the abdominal breathing verses shallow chest breathing I do hourly throughout my day.

Yoga: It is imperative to move the joints and increase blood flow no matter your condition or age. I don't recommend Bikram or Hot Yoga, especially if you're dealing with heat sensitivity. You must rehydrate with tons of water and electrolytes if you decide to try it.

Here are some basic yoga moves if you are able. Remember, no pose should be a strained effort. Do what you can comfortably.

SHIANNE LOMBARD

Yoga For Back & Neck Pain

Products: Resistance bands (these can be found on Amazon for under $20) You can travel anywhere you want with these light weight resistance bands. You can literally duplicate any exercise in the gym with these bands. Throw them in your suitcase and use them in the privacy of your hotel room.

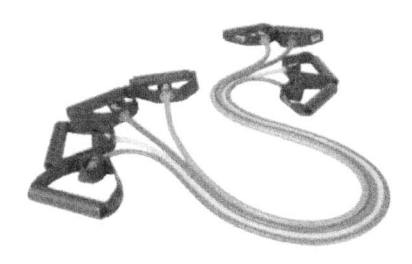

For those who suffer from **heat intolerance**: 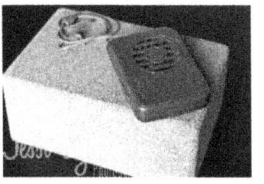 I purchased a small fan (under $10) that hangs around your neck like a necklace. It blows air up into your face and really helps keep you cool. When our internal body temperate rises, you release that heat through perspiration. In high humidity, your skin doesn't get a chance to evaporate. The fan facilitates in cooling the surface of the skin so that more heat can be released.

I also use a FitBit® for sleep. It simply tracks your restlessness at night. I look forward to waking up every morning and seeing how I slept the night before. However, remember it tracks movement and sometimes we may twitch or slightly move positions even in R.E.M. deep sleep. It tracks this as "restless sleep." So, again use it as a general gauge, but don't obsess over it.

Track Your Progress! We often forget about where we came from and how bad things really were. There are several apps online to track your symptoms, pre- and post-Cushing's, and your recovery. I highly recommend tracking everything, as it really helps us see the reality of our progress. Here are some items I used along the way.

Take pictures. Before and after pictures will really show you how far you've come.

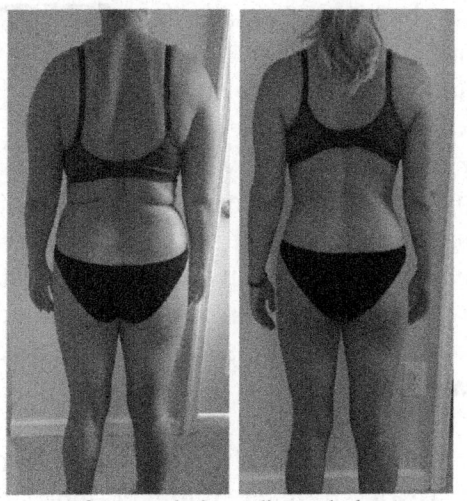

Before....and after 40lb weight loss!

My therapist recommended making a personal video about how you feel (or felt) before, during, and after surgery. I have footage moments of after I got the final diagnosis at NIH, the morning of my surgery, and several of my recovery days following surgery. Part of my personal emotional recovery was putting these onto my website for the world to see—not easy to do with the body-image hell Cushing's puts us through, but it's therapeutic in its own way, whether shared with just your loved ones or the world, or even if it's just for you.

"Like a Glove®" is a set of leggings that has a battery and unique measurement wire in the leggings. You Bluetooth it to your phone and it accurately measures as you decrease areas of your waist and hip size. Very motivating, with a progress chart and extremely accurate. I measure myself and my clients about once per month.

On the cheaper side, you could also purchase a Myotape®, which is about $10. It has a tape measure with a lock-in position to ensure accurate measurements.

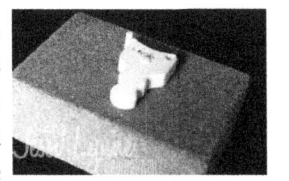

I also recommend getting a scale that also measures body fat. Tanita® scales are the best. However, I don't recommend being obsessed with the numbers on the scale—after all, we can't freak out at a device that changes 3-4lbs if you weigh in at 6am and again at 10am. It's just too variable, changing throughout the day. So, I recommend weighing in the morning before breakfast to keep it consistent. Do three days in a row and take the average of the three days. Some people recommend weighing once or twice a week. Remember that it isn't absolutely accurate with its variances, but I like that it does keep you in check so that you do not go too far in either direction, and too quickly.

Body fat is more important, and the way your clothes fit, in determining loss or gain. Tanita® can be found for around $75. You can also get body fat calipers, where you pinch your skin and it measures the thickness of fat in your midsection or different areas of the body. I use Lange® calipers, and, while the most expensive, have found them the most accurate.

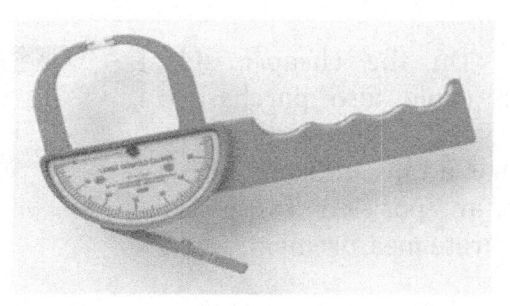

Lange body fat calipers

Concluding Thoughts

To my fellow Cushies: No matter where you are in your journey, I hope you walk away with some useful tips or at least knowing that you're not alone.

The constant running back and forth to doctors, the follow-up and re-follow up reminders for blood work and testing may seem like it will never end...**but it will.**

There is light at the end of the tunnel. Through surgeries, recoveries, and therapy. It may seem like you will never get through...**but you will**.

To gain strength both physically and emotionally, breathe. It may seem you haven't got your life back yet...**but YOU WILL.**

ABOUT THE AUTHOR

I was born in Saginaw, Michigan, where I lived until I was 12; my family then moved to Baltimore, where I stayed until my early 30s. I decided to try a new coast, and at 31 made what would be a life-changing move to San Francisco, where I met the love of my life and now husband. I loved San Francisco, it's such an amazing city, but it wasn't HOME, so we decided to settle back in Baltimore, Maryland. We have two adorable and crazy-spoiled Maltipoo puppies, Charlie and Molly, who are the joys of our lives.

When I'm not writing about my battles with Cushing's and clinical depression, I am devising exercises and fitness regimes designed specifically for those with chronic disease, and people who cannot go to a traditional personal trainer—especially one not personally experienced in the struggles with chronic illness.

You can find me through my website or Facebook page. I do in-home personal training, or at apartment gyms, and have two private studios— Sanctuary Bodyworks and Kilo Studio. I also do online Skype sessions for anyone around the world who needs help.

I would love to hear from you for feedback or your personal experiences! Be sure to visit and follow my website and blog at www.lombardfitness.com.

Most of all...thank you so much for reading my book and walking with me through my struggles!

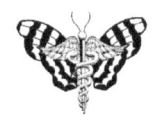

Made in the USA
Monee, IL
14 December 2020